Killing Cancer

**Fire Your Doctor
& Heal Your Body
From The Inside Out**

- Paul F. Davis -

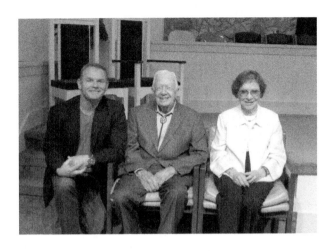

Paul with former United States President Jimmy Carter in Georgia (at 91 years of age, during which time President Carter was battling and in the process of successfully beating brain cancer) and his lovely wife Rosalynn Carter.

A Lifesaving and Life-Changing Book

- Fire Your Doctor

- Health and Wellness

- Breathe and Believe

- Detox and Eat Healthy

- Increase Oxygen

- Environmental Health

- Vitamins and Mineral Supplements

Oncologists (cancer doctors) and physicians with little education in nutrition and holistic health (and often having not completed a single course in nutrition in the medical colleges they attended, institutions heavily financed by pharmaceutical companies training doctors to embrace and push pills for profit) are going to jail throughout the United States for illegal activity and preying on patients genuinely suffering and seeking relief for physical ailments and life threatening diseases.

Doctors and pharmacists in five states in the United States (Alabama, Kentucky, Ohio, Tennessee and West Virginia) were charged in a prescription pill bust totaling 32 million pain pills. American federal prosecutors charged 60 physicians and chemists in April 2019 with illegally handing out opioid prescriptions in what they say is the biggest drug bust among medical professionals for profit of its kind in American history. As someone who has ministered to suffering cancer patients, I know firsthand the alleged "treatment" they often are receiving (by way of chemo-"therapy" and radiation) is excruciatingly painful and another opportunity for doctors to prescribe pain killers (and various other drugs, medical protocols and interventions) for profit. The joke among oncologists at dinner parties is: "The procedure was a success. The cancer is dead and gone, but so too is the patient."

Thus the militaristic approach to dealing with diseases in humans and killing pests in agriculture by using toxic, poisonous substances is greatly harming public health and the global food supply, thereby weakening human immunity, causing more cancer, and premature deaths throughout our communities.

Doctors, I am not against you, but rather I am for health and wellness. If it takes people temporarily firing their physician to enable them to take back their health and be responsible to heal their bodies from the inside out - so be it. It is time patients use doctors and stop letting doctors use patients for profit. Once patients understand the foundations of good health and wellness (body, mind and spirit); they then can be more alert, aware and proactive in cultivating a healthy lifestyle

As a survivor of substance abuse, my mother having been an alcoholic and drug addict, it saddens me to hear about prescription drug abuse (when patients entrust their lives, health and well-being to physicians who prey on them for profit and violate the Hippocratic oath to do no harm).

If you need a wellness trainer or substance abuse prevention speaker in your community or country, contact me (RevivingNations@yahoo.com)

www.PaulFDavis.com and www.EducationPro.us

www.PaulFDavis.com/substance-abuse-prevention-speaker

My book "Substance Abuse Prevention for the United States of Addiction" can be found here:

https://amzn.to/2FJCG2s

Among the doctors arrested recently in the United States, they were accused of trading drugs for sex, giving prescriptions to Facebook friends without proper medical exams and unnecessarily pulling teeth to justify writing pain pill prescriptions.

The list of indicted medical professionals includes podiatrists, orthopedic specialists, dentists, general practitioners and nurse practitioners..

Prosecutors said the specialties and methods varied among the accused, but the result in every case was the same: people addicted to pain medication received dangerous amounts of opioids, including oxycodone, methadone   and morphine.

This brings me to my question, if medical doctors and medical professionals will prescribe excessive amounts (and dosages) of pain killers for profit; what makes cancer patients think oncologists and medical doctors will not do the same with chemo-"therapy" drugs, radiation "treatment" and medical protocols and interventions to maximize their profits?

The reason I ask this is because I believe chemo-"therapy" and radiation kill the patient before the cancer will. Patients could happily live for years with cancer, but it is often very difficult to survive chemo-"therapy" and radiation (as there is nothing therapeutic about poisoning and frying your body and killing all your enzymes and good bacteria whereby your hair falls out and you feel like a walking dead person). Chemo and radiation deplete the life and vitality within the body. Surely there are better ways to kill cancer than to kill the patient along therewith.

If you think having money to finance the best medical care is the answer think again. Movie stars and famous rich people have died after having taken chemotherapy and radiation as a cancer "treatment" among whom were actor Patrick Swayze, football coach Joe Paterno, White House press secretary Tony Snow, Jackie Kennedy (wife to deceased President John F. Kennedy).

Thus there are surely better ways to treat cancer. Ask living President Jimmy Carter, who at 91 years of age beat brain cancer by refusing chemotherapy and instead opted for immunotherapy to boost his immune system and human health to combat cancer. Today President Carter, who I have personally met at his home church in Georgia where he leads Bible studies every Sunday morning is approaching 93 years of age. Prayer and faith are also powerful forces to impart supernatural life and hope to the body and heart to transcend physical ailments, illness and challenges. President Carter has many praying for and upholding him before God.

Doctors acting as drug dealers across America preying on patients for profit is a frightening state of emergency and brutal assault on public health by a highly powerful and profitable medical industry with skillful lawyers and lobbyists to protect their interests in courtrooms and the halls of government where legislation is written impacting patients and medical care protocols.

The U.S. Justice Department is calling the pushing of opioids by physicians healthcare fraud and highly irresponsible. Patients therefore should remember that every industry (medical included) is driven for profit and if the buyer (patient) is not vigilant, alert, aware and always cautious they can be taken advantage of and pay dearly financially and more importantly by way of the loss of their life (or a premature life cut short by medical malpractice or the quality of life reduced thereby).

They said the illegal prescriptions put as many as 32 million pain pills in the hands of patients. Most of the defendants face charges of unlawful distribution of controlled substances involving prescription opioids, which authorities say were given out in the magnitude and enormity of about 350,000 improper prescriptions in Alabama, Kentucky, Ohio, Tennessee, and West Virginia.

https://news.yahoo.com/news/doctors-pharmacists-5-states-charged-153853538.html?fbclid=IwAR3B38u3coHEZ9f0O MLSbBldcCFyODJyr500lNEh-orLOAqRNn5PXScB0oQ

Thank God for honest doctors who saves lives and do good. As for the other pill pushers and those recommending unnecessary surgeries for profit (like removing vital organs), here is something to consider. Perhaps many of our beloved doctors and physicians (and some pharmacists and chemists) illegibly write and sign their names because so many know the degree of their ongoing malpractice and misdiagnoses (given the American Medical Journal has itself said up to twenty-five percent of the time physicians misdiagnose) as they prey on patients for profit with prescriptions in the United States of addiction and elsewhere throughout the world and don't want to be held accountable, responsible or be tracked so easily? Psychologists and interrogators trained in lie detection have done studies on a person's signature to reveal aspects about their personality and professionalism.

This being said and considering some oncologists have reported cancer doctors can earn up to $250,000 a year in medical insurance payments to "treat" one cancer patient; there is a financial incentive for physicians working with cancer patients to keep them weak, needy and coming back for more "treatments" so they can "get it" (get all their money, or the money via their insurers; excuse me I meant get all the cancer in order to give the patient a clean bill of health). Perhaps the motive of physicians is both, but if patients have a holistic alternative to kill cancer and live stronger, why are physicians pushing poisonous protocols, toxic drugs and deadly radiation? When will Congress mandate and legislate prison time for physicians preying on patients for profit and not telling them all of their available options (medical versus holistic) to treat deadly diseases such as cancer?

Model Guidelines for the Use of Complementary and Alternative Therapies in Medical Practice

https://www.ncbi.nlm.nih.gov/books/NBK83798/

"CAM" Education in Medical Schools: A Critical Opportunity Missed - AMA Journal of Ethics

https://journalofethics.ama-assn.org/article/cam-education-medical-schools-critical-opportunity-missed/2011-06

Integrative Medicine and Cancer Care - AMA Journal of Ethics

https://journalofethics.ama-assn.org/article/integrative-medicine-and-cancer-care/2011-06

"Over the past decade, CAM practices have become even more popular, especially among individuals with chronic diseases such as cancer. ...Unfortunately, the term "CAM" causes consternation among many of our professional colleagues who perceive that their patients are forgoing conventional therapy" (Integrative Medicine and Cancer Care).

Afraid they may lose business when patients catch on to the medical industry's for profit racket and stop trusting physicians; the American Medical Association has stopped using terminology such as alternative and holistic medicine (lest they be replaced and become irrelevant) and instead are opting to use words like "complementary" and "integrative" to ensure conventional medicine still has a role to play in patients' lives. When medical reform fully takes place in years to come, patients will be permitted to use their health and medical insurance to pay for holistic health and alternative medicine and no longer be bound and forced (financially incentivized) to opt for conventional medicine, the latter of which often does not work and comes with harmful side effects or unnecessary invasive procedures or surgeries that never deal with the root of the problem internally. Chemo-"therapy" is a euphemism and misnomer, a failed medical practice for more than 50 years. Any alleged "success stories" are questionable, because cancer can easily be cured from the inside out with lifestyle changes, diet, healthy and natural remedies without the toxic poison used in chemo-"therapy" that weakens human immunity and nearly kills patients (sometimes killing both the cancer and the patient as already mentioned by name in this book). Useless, unnecessary and invasive conventional medical practices; like testicular removal for elderly men with prostate cancer kill the medical industry's credibility (and that of their toothless regulatory bodies allowing them to get away with harming humans and committing murder, ongoing crimes against humanity for profit). The medical industry must publicly acknowledge their failures, stop these procedures, and move on to new alternative forms of treatment (even if that costs them financially). Otherwise if not, the medical industry and physicians will lose all public trust and patients' dollars entirely.

"Many leading cancer centers have established integrative medicine programs where complementary therapies such as acupuncture, massage therapy, nutrition counseling, physical activity, and stress management techniques are offered alongside conventional cancer therapies. These programs often provide guidance to patients in choosing the most safe and effective CAM therapies to incorporate into their plan of care.

There is an increasing body of research on the benefits of many CAM practices. Studies provide evidence that some integrative therapies benefit cancer patients by improving their quality of life and reducing disease symptoms and treatment side effects" (Integrative Medicine and Cancer Care).

Since the conventional chemo-"therapy" is so deadly, toxic, painful and full of harmful side effects, it is only fair that "patients have a right to explore all health care options" and it is physicians "responsibility to help guide them through their decision-making process" (Integrative Medicine and Cancer Care) and not guide then in a self-serving way to enrich the physician financially, but truly provide a full array of all available options and the accompany side effects of each. Calling CAM controversial is ridiculous compared to the enormity of harm caused by chem-"therapy" and radiation to the human body, often devastating human immunity and resulting in death. These doctors of death therefore must be sued by patients and their families until medical reform brings about change throughout the medical industry. Unfortunately, few in any industry for profit see the light and do the right thing until they first feel the heat.

Decisions to Use Complementary and Alternative Medicine (CAM) by Male Cancer Patients: Information-Seeking Roles and Types of Evidence Used

https://www.ncbi.nlm.nih.gov/pmc/articles/PMC20 00907/

"Complementary and Alternative Medicine (CAM) is increasingly popular with cancer patients and yet information provision or discussion about CAM by health professionals remains low. Previous research suggests that patients may fear clinicians' 'disapproval' if they raise the subject of CAM, and turn to other sources to acquire information about CAM."

The irony is so many are terrified and afraid of cancer, but few patients ever slow down long enough to ask their doctor a few simple questions to assist them in ridding their body of cancer:

1. What does cancer look like in shape, appearance, texture and color?

2. What is the cause of cancer?

3. What can I do to remove cancer from my body?

Sadly most patients quietly relinquish all control of their health to doctors and physicians, the latter of which quite frankly may not know the answers to these questions, nor have they taken the time to inquire and find out (in order to genuinely be able to help their patients).

My dermatologist at Spring Street Derm in Soho, Manhattan was hesitant when I asked about natural cures to say anything (possibly because she feared losing a paying patient and secondly getting in trouble with the American Medical Association that protects the profitable medical industry and discourages alternative medicine in practice).

Yet the American Medical Association does say on their website physicians are required and obligated to advise and inform their patients of available alternative holistic health options and not only push the medical and pharmaceutical paradigm. However in my experience, I have yet to see a physician who does so (as pushing the medical approach is far more profitable for physicians personally).

Patients should unite and initiate a class action lawsuit against physicians and doctors who fail to recommend holistic health options and alternatives to medicine and invasive surgeries. Here below are some interesting articles and official codes of conduct for physicians and doctors.

Complementary and Alternative Medicine - Canadian Medical Association (CMA) Policy

"...decisions about health care interventions used in Canada should be based on sound scientific evidence as to their safety, efficacy and effectiveness - the same standard by which physicians and all other elements of the health care system should be assessed. Patients deserve the highest standard of treatment available, and physicians, other health practitioners, manufacturers, regulators and researchers should all work toward this end. All elements of the health care system should "consider first the well-being of the patient."

The ethical principle of non-maleficence obliges physicians to reduce their patient's risks of harm. Physicians must constantly strive to balance the potential benefits of an intervention against its potential side effects, harms or burdens. To help physicians meet this obligation, patients should inform their physician if the patient uses CAM."

https://policybase.cma.ca/documents/policypdf/PD1 5-09.pdf

In America, all the TV commercials tell patients to: "Ask your doctor...." Yet the Canadian Medical Association code of ethics tells patients to "inform their doctor" if they use complementary and alternative medicine (CAM) approaches to health and wellness. Thus patients must be more proactive and stop relinquishing control of their health and well-being to physicians and doctors who typically are inclined to pursue the profitable approach to enrich themselves first (be it interventions and invasive surgeries, pharmaceutical prescriptions, expensive diagnostic and thorough evaluative tests, etc.). Nevertheless the Hippocratic oath tells physicians to "do no harm," but in practice in this medical industry age for profit; if it is legally permitted, doctors see their practice as committing

no harm (despite other more holistic, sustainable

and inexpensive options being available to patients).

Model Guidelines for the Use of Complementary

and Alternative Therapies in Medical Practice

Approved by the House of Delegates

of the Federation of State Medical Boards (FSMB)

of the United States, as policy April 2002

https://www.fsmb.org/siteassets/advocacy/policies/
model-guidelines-for-the-use-of-complementary-
and-alternative-therapies-in-medical-practice.pdf

"Physicians, indeed all health-care professionals,

have a duty not only to avoid harm but also a

positive duty to do good— that is, to act in the

patient's best interest[s]. This duty of beneficence takes precedence over any self-interest."

The above quote from the policy of the FSMB is written and clearly stated (and necessary) because this regulatory body knows damn good and well that all physicians do not put the patient's interest over and before their own in all of their decision-making, prescriptions, and the medical advice they render to patients. Otherwise this statement would not need to be mentioned (and written at the beginning of their "model guidelines for medical practice").

One thing I respect about Chinese acupuncture is their "medicine" is nothing more than naturally occurring herbs and substances (nothing chemically concocted in laboratory, but rather substance your body can easily process and more readily absorb). Moreover Chinese medicine has been around for thousands of years, China having one of the longest living civilizations. Nevertheless I'm sure like most physicians there are some acupuncturists who sell fear, doing and saying whatever they deem will keep the patient coming back for more treatments.

However in praise and defense of Chinese acupuncture I will tell you a personal story and testimony. One afternoon my ex-wife (Canadian) and I were walking around Lake Eola in Orlando, Florida. There were various tables and booths erected alongside the sidewalk promoting their food, products and services.

We saw one man conducting exams on people with a small device that traced along their ear. It caught my attention, so I stopped to watch. The Chinese acupuncturist after a minute or two would tell the person what was wrong with them physically and point out areas of weakness within their bodies.

Being the hesitant skeptic and curious childlike adult I am; I was fascinated and intrigued to see if this actually worked. The Chinese acupuncturist and his assistant showed me a printed diagram of the ear, which visually pointed out the ear is precisely the shape of a fetus in the womb of a mother and therefore somewhat of a smaller grid to the meridians and critical areas (organs) of the body; whereby complications and problem areas could be identified.

As a believer in God, I was in awe and began to smile; convinced this seemed like the Creator to hide a roadmap to the human body on the ear externally (which few have discovered, uncovered or examined). Upon examining my ex-wife with the device, the acupuncturist told her that her problems existed in her lower abdomen (female organs area). I was shocked, as in fact we had difficulty having sex for a couple years due to her always being in pain. My ex-wife got teary eyed and was in awe of the accuracy of the Chinese acupuncturist. As for me, he identified some pain in my lower back, which indeed was due to dehydration, me taking too many body building supplements and not drinking enough water (of course he did not know the exact reason for my lower back pain within my kidney).

When I visited an Acupuncturist College for a few years and allowed graduates to practice on me, I was impressed how detailed their inquiry was and questions they would ask (interviewing me for 30 to 45 minutes before ever doing anything on my body, before which they consulted their supervisor and masters of studies to inquire further before proceeding).

This is how modern medicine should be practiced. However the medicine for profit paradigm, which I have experienced all of my life in the United States, puts patients in several waiting rooms before they see a general family practice doctor, and then suddenly the physician appears to interact with the patient for 5 minutes or less, after which the patient is sent to the bill collector and made to pay between $150 to $300, obtain his or her prescription, and run to the pharmacy to get their drugs.

Should the patient be healthy and not return annually or every two or three years to see the doctor; the clinic will often refuse them any complimentary service (such as the nurse's signature on a tuberculosis test county school boards require teachers to obtain). The family medical clinic I visited for over 30 years with my grandparents refused to sign my simple tuberculosis document for the local school board saying, "Sorry, you have not been here for a few years and we can't do that until you see the doctor."

I laughed and said, "I'm not sick. Why should I see the doctor?" Of course I knew it was all about making money for this medical clinic, walked out and never returned. I drove a couple blocks down the road to another medical clinic I had never before visited, caught a nurse walking down the hall, asked her to sign the school board document, which she did, and I was never asked to pay a penny.

Such is the way medicine, physicians' practices, and clinics operate often in America. Thank God for the good hearted people in the medical industry, clinics and hospitals. The rest of them need to have a close encounter with an angry and frustrated father figure like John Q and widespread public protestation demanding reform of this corrupt and evil medical industry denying patients care and treatment when needed lest they can pay for it.

The movie John Q (played by Denzel Washington) is definitely worth watching. Check it out here: https://amzn.to/2V6m4KR

Health Advice

Undoubtedly good nutrition, a healthy lifestyle, and supporting your body with the right vitamins, minerals and enzymes; will fortify your immune system to combat and prevent many deadly diseases including cancer. If you want to live stronger and longer that will not be facilitated by spending hours every week visiting your doctor, but by taking back your health and becoming educated to live a healthy lifestyle. Imagine how much you could do and accomplish if you were physically stronger, mentally clearer and sharper, and able to achieve personal peak performance to live optimally spirit, mind and body.

Although I am not a medical doctor (thank God for that), I am a former lifeguard, personal fitness trainer, wellness trainer, and nutritional consultant. Remember medical doctors are trained in medical schools, which are heavily financed by pharmaceutical companies (their chief financiers which heavily lean on and influence medical schools to advocate a pill pushing paradigm that enriches drug companies rather than advocating and suggesting alternative medicine and holistic health remedies that truly benefit patients and make them healthy and not likely to return as frequently to see doctors).

For legal purposes to cover my ass, like all others writing health books, I will tell you (although I myself don't believe it and certainly would never take this advice when seeking HEALTH); "ask your doctor" before doing anything. However you also may want to read "Dead Doctors Don't Lie"

(http://amzn.to/1q7BBGy) written by one brilliant medical doctor who compiled obituaries when doctors died and thereby proved doctors are not as smart as we think and error when caring for their own health. I know this to be true, because my grandmother's doctor smoked (and smoked so much I could be smell it on him, as his nurse confirmed with embarrassment when I asked).

The New York Times, Newsweek, and other reputable news sources have themselves written articles on the questionable ties of medical colleges with pharmaceutical companies (even to the extent of giving Harvard a D and near failing marks for ethics violations in taking pharmaceutical money and allowing it to influence the medical college students' curriculum).

Furthermore many universities professors write in journals that are funded by pharmaceutical companies to achieve preordained conclusions (to favor the creation of a new drug, support the use of a drug, and increase the sales of a drug) to support the pharmaceutical industry and perpetuate their existence, not the furtherance of good health in humans as promised when physicians take a Hippocratic oath to obtain their medical license (because in the medical industry ongoing sickness is the money maker, not health). Thus the medical, psychiatric and pharmaceutical industries all thrive on creating new diseases, names for these diseases, keeping patients sick (but hopeful to improve) and thereafter creating new drugs to allegedly (though with multiple side affects) "cure" the problem (or dismantle the synergy and total wellness of the human body, by disrupting the body's immunity and connected inter-reliance to thereby ensure ongoing patient illness and sickness - thus making them a profitable patient for life).

Nevertheless since some will not believe me, I suggest reading a book written by a medical doctor and professor at Harvard Medical College on "How Doctors Think" (http://amzn.to/1k7ShMP), which acknowledges as reported by the American Journal of Medicine that doctors error in their diagnoses of patients up to 25% of the time.

Fire Your Doctor

When I met President Jimmy Carter at his home church in Georgia, not far from where he was a peanut farmer before he got involved in politics, President Carter was 91 years young at that time. Jimmy was fighting brain cancer, which many predicted would kill him at that age.

Yet President Carter was smarter than most patients because he did not allow doctors and physicians using chemotherapy and radiation to attack, invade and destroy his body (all to destroy some cancer in the brain simultaneously). Instead President Carter wisely took a holistic approach to health, employing immunotherapy to strengthen his body's immune system to fight the cancer (a concerted, holistic effort unlike chemo that wipes out and destroys the human immune system, causing hair fallout and many other deadly consequences that kills many people).

The list of patients killed by chemotherapy and radiation is endless ranging from Jackie Kennedy Onassis (the former president's wife), Patrick Swayze (actor), Joe Paterno (football coach) and Tony Snow (White House press secretary). All of these wonderful people are now dead (as are many others) thanks to chemo "therapy" (a euphemism and misnomer as there is nothing therapeutic about chemo and radiation) and radiation destroying their body's defense and offense mechanisms to fight off diseases and sustain good health internally. Thus the joke among oncologists and cancer doctors at parties is, "The operation was a success. The cancer is gone and the patient is dead."

If prematurely dying is your goal, then by all means listen to all your doctor says about cancer and be one of the many patients who enriches doctors $250,000 annually to be "treated" for cancer (and possibly killed in the process).

Health and Wellness

Clearly health and wellness has little to do with practicing medicine, because so few medical schools teach nutrition (being heavily financed by drug companies to push pills for profit rather than health for patients well-being, lest they lose clients visiting their clinic and medical establishment for profit).

When people become proactive about their health, read the labels of the food they buy at the grocery store (preferably before purchasing and consuming the product, not after they get home, although returning less than healthy products is also advisable to send a message to food manufacturers to clean up their ingredients or pay the consequences), and make healthy choices; they live stronger and longer.

Ignorant and duped consumers buy "food" based on colorful packaging and adverts, like when I was a small child and saw a cool cartoon and ran to my grandmother asking her to buy the cereal as advertised for me. Although she did, today in retrospect I think I probably would have grown taller and been bigger had I not eaten so many sugar filled cereals and treats as a youngster growing up.

Nevertheless today I make smart and educated food choices for myself and my daughter.

Detox and Eat Healthy

Among the many ways to detox is to consume cruciferous vegetables (or powder) which cleanses and scrubs the digestive tract, removing Candida (fungus in slimy liquid form), cancer and other obtrusive blockages getting in the way from fluid bowel movements, food processing, assimilation and elimination of waste.

Primary greens is one powder I like to take in the morning with some juice (pick your personal favorite) to cleanse the digestive system when beginning the day. It will help improve regularity, remove toxic metals and other substances polluting the body. Remember 60% or more of the human immune system is in the gut (the intestines).

Among my favorite powerful greens blends to energize your body, cleanse your intestines and remove toxins and heavy metals are:

- Garden of Life Raw Organic Perfect Food: 100% USA Organic Wheat Grass Juice - Vegan, Gluten Free Whole Food Supplement

https://amzn.to/2FL0uWP

- Garden of Life Whole Food Fruit and Vegetable

Supplement - Perfect Food Superfood Green

Dietary Powder Berry, 240g

https://amzn.to/2FGcwzu

- Garden of Life Raw Organic Perfect Food
Energizer Juiced Green Superfood Greens Powder -
Yerba Mate, Pomegranate - Vegan Gluten Free
Whole Food Dietary Supplement, Plus Probiotics

https://amzn.to/2TKDSts

- Garden of Life Greens and Protein Powder -

Organic Raw Protein and Greens with

Probiotics/Enzymes, Vegan, Gluten-Free, Vanilla,

19.3oz (1lb 3 oz/548g) Powder

https://amzn.to/2U6tReX

- Garden of Life Organic Protein Powder - Vegan Plant-Based Protein Powder, Chocolate, 9.7oz (276g) Powder

https://amzn.to/2HOOeqJ

- Garden of Life Meal Replacement - Organic Raw Plant Based Protein Powder, Lightly Sweet, Vegan, Gluten-Free, 36.6oz (2lb 5oz/1,038g) Powder

https://amzn.to/2V6uEsM

- Garden of Life Raw Organic Perfect Food Alkalizer & Detoxifier Juiced Greens Superfood Powder - Lemon Ginger, 30 Servings - Non-GMO, Gluten Free Whole Food Dietary Supplement, Plus Probiotics

https://amzn.to/2FF6BL5

- Pure Hawaiian Spirulina Green Complete Superfood Powder– Vegan, Non GMO – Natural Superfood Grown in Hawaii

https://amzn.to/2CMWL9w

- Berry Green Superfood with Goji, Acai & Raspberry, Raw Organic Nutrition- Vegan & Gluten Free - 240 Grams

https://amzn.to/2V4xDCh

Beyond vegetables and their detoxifying fiber, I want to share some of my favorite foods that are bitter and burn.

Blessing in That Which is Bitter or Burns

Citrus and other fruit rich in vitamin C is very useful to scrub, cleanse and detoxify the digestive tract and energize the immune system to fight and combat free radicals in the body. I particularly like to use organic lemons in fruit smoothies. I mention organic lemons because then after rinsing them with warm water, I can cut up the entire lemon with the skin (peel) thereon. If the lemons are not organic, anticipate they are heavily sprayed with pesticides and herbicides, which I recommend not to eat (that being the outside peel). Non-organic lemons (or citrus) remove the peel when eating, blending or juicing.

Of course this can be a bitter experience, but an energizing one indeed. Therefore to balance the bitterness one of my favorite concoctions is organic apple juice (not from concentrate) and an organic lemon. The apple juice is quite sweet, which the lemon goes well with (in my opinion). You can find the amount and portion size that works for you. Sometimes you may want to start with half or a quarter of a lemon until you get used to it.

The apple juice helps open your bile ducts to remove liver and gallbladder stones and the lemon simultaneously will be a powerful detox agent to fight cancer. In my experience, usually within an hour of this apple and lemon smoothie I'm running to the toilet to take care of business as my intestines get liberated and cleansed of some excess lingering around that needs to move on.

Other beneficial bitter things I enjoy that also burn are garlic and ginger. Garlic saved my life in southeast Asia when I traveled through some impoverished places as a missionary and found myself with pain in my lower back (kidney area). This was long before I became a health nut when I was eating almost anything and everything. The primary culprit and contaminant however was bad water or poor hygiene among the locals preparing my food in places like Africa, India, Thailand, Myanmar, Malaysia and Indonesia. Eventually I got smart and ate less meat (or smaller animals which were less prone to be butchered and sit in the hot sun get contaminated or infested with flies all day waiting for someone to buy or cook them). Dried fish in the sun with flies and maggots thereon was something I only had to endure once (coming out the next morning from both sides) to ensure I never ate fish again (now knowing where it came from and how villagers prepared and where they purchased it). I don't enjoy vomiting and diarrhea.

Again I was a missionary in some very remote places without refrigeration and free flowing water. Thus "road runner" (chicken), a smaller animal, more easy to kill, sell and consume in full (and less likely to sit around with multiplying bacteria and flies landing on it) became my go to meat and protein source.

Larger animals as I mentioned when out in the villages in remote places can take a long time to consume and while waiting from the time of slaughter to purchase to transport home to refrigeration are more susceptible to contamination. Thus my eventual quote when asked what I like to eat: "Fruit, vegetables, rice, bread, eggs and chicken - chicken is my friend."

When after having typhoid in Myanmar and Thailand, I began eating a wedge of raw garlic (from an entire clove) daily (either with bread or my meal), which I found alleviated lower back pain (and internal discomfort in my kidneys from drinking foul water and eating food that disagreed with me).

I once had left a clove of garlic in my backpack while traveling by train from south to north India and back, which I later discovered two months later and to my shock and surprise; there was no mold or decay of the garlic. It was then I realized what a powerful antioxidant and immune builder garlic truly is (as any other produce, fruit or vegetables would have begun to rot in days and decayed).

Ginger is another thing that burns that works wonderfully to aid digestion, strengthen the body's immunity and rid the body of toxins. It's ironic, saddening and sickening that medical doctors (who rarely take a single course in nutrition in medical college) fail to mention these immune boosting natural substances to patients so they instead can push profitable pills (medicine) that significantly disrupts human immunity and have harmful side effects (many medicines polluting the body's liver and kidneys).

Ginger stimulates heat and circulation in the body, the burning effect I mentioned, which kills diseases. When I get a fever (rarely), it is often accompanied by chills. By simply bundling up under the blankets I quickly sweat it out and the heat in my body breaks the fever (often in 6 to 12 hours, or less).

Dr. Hiromi Shinya, medical doctor and professor at Einstein Medical College (author of "The Enzyme Factor") says heat in the body stimulates the movement of enzymes. Enzymes are vitally important to move and transport vitamins and minerals throughout the body to do their important work including combat viruses and diseases.

Thus fewer people get sick during spring and summer in warmer climates. This explains why many elderly (who typically tend to get more cold in their bodies as they age and enzymes are depleted and in decline) often seek to live in Florida the sunshine state (my home state where I was born).

In Chinese health and acupuncture they have something called "Chinese bitters" which I have not before used, but once again I am indeed a believer in bitters and that which burns. Even here in southeast Asia where I am now living, I recently spoke to someone regarding dengue fever and was told they eat a spicy soup with hot chili peppers if ever they or a loved one gets dengue fever. Filipinos say the spicy hot soup kills dengue on the spot and removes the parasitic infection and deadly disease. Thus God our Creator has put things in the earth to fortify our immunity and enable us to thrive and overcome the parasites, animal viruses, environmental elements and physical challenges we face while living on the planet. In fact the Bible declares "the leaves of the tree of life" in eternity will provide "healing for the nations" (Revelation 22:1-2). Spiritual things mirror natural things (1Corinthians 11:14), the supernatural beginning with the foundational word "natural." Thus God indeed has put things on earth to help humanity survive and thrive physically, be in health, happy, strong and at peace.

Grapefruit and oranges are acidic, a bit less bitter than lemons, but equally useful and rich in vitamin C to strengthen the body's immunity and combat cancer.

Fruit is rich in glutathione the precursor to all energy in the body. Thus I eat a lot of raw fruit daily to provide immediate fuel and energy to the body. Marathon runners and triathlon athletes consume a lot of fruit for immediate energy, realizing the body can quickly process, digest, absorb, and assimilate this energy source (unlike meat protein that takes up to 8 hours or more to digest and eliminate depending on the quality of the cut of meat and the way it is cooked).

Tropical climates have a fruit called Soursop that is said to be anti-cancerous and able to rid the body of cancer. Soursop is the fruit of Annona muricata, a broadleaf, flowering, evergreen tree. The exact origin is unknown; it is native to the tropical regions of the Americas, the Caribbean and some parts of Asia.

I have tasted soursop before in the Philippines and find it to be quite refreshing. Since cancer thrives on sugar in the body, which is why I often liken cancer to Candida (like the sugary lactose flem found in the mouth and throat after drinking milk), bitter fruits that burn are very helpful to cut through the Candida and cancerous substances (undigested proteins) in the body.

Another fruit I recently learned of from friends in the Philippines (that grows in west Africa) is what is known as "miracle fruit" because the berry of the fruit is used as medicine to treat diabetes and correct the imbalances in the body caused by cancer and chemotherapy. Apparently chemotherapy causes taste disturbances. Miracle fruit is also used as a low calorie sugar free sweetener.

As known throughout generations, mothers have used lemon oil and other citrus blends for household cleaning to remove dirt, grime, gunk and cut through the grease when scrubbing pots and pans after cooking. The same applies with lemons, citrus, garlic and ginger when cleaning your intestines and body from the inside out. Moreover great chefs know how to balance the acidity and sweetness when cooking. This is why ginger is often used with beef in China, or lemongrass in soups throughout Thailand (often using coconut milk, which is antifungal and antibacterial in its properties).

Although I have traveled to 89 nations thus far at the writing of this book, there are so many more healthy natural remedies to heal the body that I have yet to discover. I would be delighted to hear from you and appreciate your insights as to what has worked for you (especially that which burns and is better in the earth and your native health remedies). I realize this book has only begun to scratch the surface, but surely it will help you to think more holistically and pursue balance in the body.

After years of eating ice-cream and sweets from our childhood into adulthood, it only makes sense our bodies need some bitters and things that burn to reverse the harmful cancerous effects of excessive sugar in the body and undigested protein lingering in the digestive tract causing putrid odors and toxic substances to multiply and spread. This explains why people manifest unsightly sores and spots on their skin, as their body seeks to cleanse the toxins within and push them through the epidermis to find relief.

Sunlight and Detoxification

Thankfully 20 minutes a day in the sun with exposure to vitamin D will help the skin accelerate the detoxification process. Although some will claim the sun causes cancer, I wholeheartedly disagree. First of all, if the sun was so toxic, why would God Almighty put the sun in the center of the universe to energize and provide life to all planets and living things? Remember the earth revolves around the sun, without which there would be no photosynthesis and fruit and vegetables to eat. Moreover oncologists (cancer doctors) tell us among all the important vitamins to combat cancer, vitamin D is number one (the sun providing humans free vitamin D daily if we will just take our clothes off and get outdoors more often).

Another interesting rebuttal to those who contend the sun causes cancer is if this is so, why do so many cancerous growth on the skin occur in places least exposed to the sun? Such as the back of a person? Why not their arms or forehead? I believe it is because cancer is merely an outward manifestation of what is already occurring within the body. Our skin is just trying to help detoxify our organs internally to excrete and remove foul substances within as we sweat, come in contact with the sun, saunas, heat and any other way we can stimulate circulation in the body (including exercise and sexercise). Circulation and sweating is good for you, Do more of it. Turn off the television and computer. Get outdoors and start moving!

Breathe and Believe

When I traveled and ministered in Papua New Guinea, an 11 year old girl attended the church meeting. When I had an altar call for salvation, inviting people to give their lives to Christ, many surrendered their hearts to Jesus. Thereafter I prayed for those sick in body.

While praying for the sick, an 11 year old young girl (who I had never seen before, nor interacted with, and knew nothing about) had a demonic reaction the moment I looked at her. She began screaming, "I hate you!"

Knowing this was not the young girl, but the demon in her; I began laughing and replied, "I hate you too devil; now come out of her in Jesus Name!" That night the young girl was set free. I also led her in a prayer to forgive her parents, after learning she was adopted and had anger, bitterness and resentment toward her parents for abandoning her and putting her up for adoption.

As a result of casting out the demon causing the anger and bitterness (Matthew 8:16), upon returning home to the United States, I received a personal hand written letter from the young girl in Papua New Guinea sharing her testimony. She said not only was she delivered from a tormenting evil spirit and unforgiveness toward her parents the night I prayed for her; but she also was thereafter healed of asthma.

This is precisely how the ministry of Jesus operated. When Christ set the captives free tormented and vexed by demon spirits, often times thereafter they were instantly healed and made well physically. Upon liberating those "oppressed by the devil;" Jesus was able to restore divine health to people so they could be whole body-mind-spirit (see Acts 10:38; Matthew 8:16).

Jesus Christ is the same yesterday, today, and forever (Hebrews 13:8); as I myself have witnessed in Papua New Guinea with the precious orphan girl and in countless other situations throughout the world when I prayed for people in the mighty and merciful Name of Jesus, during which the miracle working Holy Spirit showed up and showed off the power of God to save, heal and deliver humanity without controversy, dispute or contradiction (Hebrews 2:4).

The Holy Spirit that rose Jesus Christ from the dead following His crucifixion on the cross for the sins of humanity, is mighty to save, heal and deliver humanity still today and forevermore for whosoever believes and dares to receive (see Romans 8:11; John 11:40).

I realize some will be skeptical, as I myself was when I first attended Pastor Benny Hinn's church in Orlando, Florida years ago. However once I felt the "Supernatural Fire" of God in me and on my body (in a youth service wherein Pastor Benny was not present and no human touched me physically, I realized it was God's electrifying and arresting Presence and not about a man or personality), as thoroughly shared in my personal testimony and book available here (https://amzn.to/2OmGzif), wherein Biblical holy Scriptures are cited throughout the book to confirm and prove God's will, intent, supernatural ways, and how our Creator heals and deals with humanity throughout history.

Science recognizes electromagnetic therapy as capable of killing parasites and healing the body. In fact there are people in the health and wellness sector who sell "zappers" for over $2,000 US dollars online to use electromagnetic pulses to kill parasites. I have never used them however because I know the Bible says the fire of the Holy Spirit will burn away the chaff in our lives and our God is a consuming fire (see Luke 3:16-17; Hebrews 12:19). Thus I rest in peace knowing when I connect with God in worship and praise, as I have countless times, I can feel the supernatural fire of Almighty God that will heal me body, mind and spirit and make me whole and complete in Christ (Colossians 2:10). Nevertheless "according to your faith, be it unto you" (Matthew 9:29), because it is impossible to please God without faith (Hebrews 11:6) the currency of heaven. He who doubts is damned already (Romans 14:23).

The breathe of life ultimately comes from God (Genesis 2:7) in whom we live, move and have our being (Acts 17:28). Job wrote and said, "The Spirit of God has made me, and the breathe of the Almighty has given me life" (Job 33:4). Thus Job recognized God's Holy Spirit not only gives us life (Job 27:3) and forms us in our mother's womb (Ecclesiastes 11:5), but after birth sustains us throughout our lives as well.

As a former lifeguard working in pools and on a lake at a public park, I know very well that swimmers cannot last more than 2 minutes without oxygen. It is no different for humans on dry land. Oxygen and blood flow is vital for bodily circulation and sustaining life.

Yet most emphases related to health and fitness tend to focus on exercise and ignore diet, maximizing oxygen intake and minimizing stress. Dr. Oz, a heart surgeon and Oprah's doctor, has often said stress is the number one killer. If that is true, than we need to try to reduce and minimize our stress.

As I discovered when enduring a brutal divorce and going through a painful transition, my mental and emotional state was going through turbulence which manifested in the form of a shingles virus in my body (leaving me bed ridden for nearly a month as it felt as if my internal organs had been beaten by a baseball bat and as if my skin externally had been burned by a blow torch). Shingles is indeed no joke, nor a laughing matter, but quite painful.

I spoke to the nurse at the emergency room, who informed me her sister got shingles during her divorce. Then a lady working at Home Depot during my checkout when paying for items also confirmed she too had shingles during a divorce. Thus mental and emotional stress can trigger a physical breakdown within the body. Therefore it is important for us to stay away (or at least minimize interactions with) from people who annoy, aggravate and stress us out (as much as possible).

When people are under stress and anxiety, they are more inclined to breathe shallow and take in less oxygen. Being restricted emotionally and neurologically within results in changes in a person's breathing, typically their breathing becoming more shallow, cautious, and less free flowing.

I understand breathing problems personally because when I was born, I was put in an oxygen tent for the first month of my life, as I had pneumonia and nearly died.

As the documentary film, "The Business of Being Born" reveals,

http://amzn.to/2eUk1DN

modern medicine is such that physicians and hospitals prey on patients to increase their profit margins (which sometimes involves unnecessary "interventions" to speed up the delivery, ease the doctor's workload, take the mother out of the picture via sedation, and thereafter let the doctor take control). Of course none of these approaches is good for the baby's health, nor the mother's (all the while severing the vitally important physical and emotional connection between the mother and baby).

In Africa, mothers give birth to their babies squatting and work with gravity so the baby drops and comes out nicely. One woman in Mozambique (in the middle of a treacherous storm) years ago, even gave birth in a tree (as CNN reported). Thus giving birth without the assistance and nearby presence of medical doctors happens every day throughout Africa and many developing countries where I have traveled and lived.

The opposite occurs in the western world where the physician's comfort is the primary focus, which results in pregnant mothers being laid on their backs on an elevated table so doctors can easily access and "deliver" the baby. The only problem is natural child births sometimes can last many hours (as I discovered when my daughter was born under water in a Jacuzzi at a birth center with no doctors present - a beautiful and peaceful process that lasted 12 hours or more).

The midwife and doula were very kind, encouraging, patient and supportive. My ex-wife laid in the warm Jacuzzi resting and waiting. She only agonized right at the point of delivery, after which the joy of our daughter's birth filled us with incredible peace and emotional release.

I can only wish my own birth was as painless, glorious and free from medical intrusions and interference. Unfortunately, my mother was a smoker and likely slipped up a bit during her pregnancy, which quite possibly may have resulted in me nearly suffocating in the womb with pneumonia. Under this circumstance, the presence of medical doctors proved necessary and helpful (as I was put in an oxygen tent). Yet there is a possibility that my mother did not smoke during her pregnancy (as my father thinks she did not) and a medical intervention of some sort damaged my lung or lungs temporarily giving me pneumonia.

One thing is for certain, many pregnant young ladies who drink alcohol and smoke do not discover they are pregnant until a month or more into the pregnancy (all the while negatively impacting their baby's health with their consumption of alcohol and tobacco). Quite possible this can be much more fatal and deadly during the first month or two of pregnancy. Thus birth defects can be caused sometimes by substance abuse on the part of the parents. Yes, even the father's use of harmful substances impacts the child.

I cannot ask my mother today regarding this because she was killed by an 18 year old drunk driver. My father now has Alzheimer's and is getting up there in years.

Yet my studies of health and nutrition, as someone who has earned Master degrees in Health (University of Alabama) and Global Food Law (Michigan State College of Law) taught me about the problems with the American Medical Industry (an industry for profit, not truly motivated to serve people - as I personally have repeatedly experienced whenever I visited medical clinics, doctors offices, or hospitals in the United States and was asked for my social security number, credit card billing information, address, and to sign a stack of legal documents to ensure I paid for the visit; long before I ever saw or spoke to a doctor).

In fact often times the outdated medical drugs prescribed by doctors in the USA have horrible side effects resulting in death (such a Vioxx - a drug originally intended to treat arthritis created by Merck that killed over 500,000 people giving them heart attacks).

The devastating effect of Merck's drug Vioxx preying on the elderly (and exacerbating their arthritis as the body excretes calcium from the bones to remove such toxic drugs from the body) was evident throughout America because the year the toxic drug was introduced and went to market in 1999, this year showed the largest rise in the American death rate. Conversely, in 2004, when Vioxx was pulled from the drug market and kept from consumers, the death rate in America substantially declined. Thus Americans are often being killed by their pill pushing physicians for profit. Later studies by the United States Food and Drug Administration (FDA) proved that the use of Vioxx led to deaths from cardiovascular diseases such as heart attacks and strokes, reminding us all of the painful and deadly side effects of drugs (one claimed to solve one ailment, while causing several more, and in this case resulting in death).

https://www.legalexaminer.com/health/vioxx-killed-half-a-million-the-facts-are-grim/

https://www.theweek.co.uk/us/46535/when-half-million-americans-died-and-nobody-noticed

https://www.theamericanconservative.com/articles/chinese-melamine-and-american-vioxx-a-comparison/

It is therefore worth remembering that drugs are toxic, come with harmful side effects, and are often deadly (some "working" and delivering death more speedily than others). Therefore a holistic approach to health must be pursued by consumers and patients to avoid the deadly practices of physicians for profit seeking to prey on patients and monetize the moment.

Even antibiotics have now been eclipsed by morphing bacteria that now are becoming stronger and smarter than antibiotics. In fact most "super bugs" (viruses and infectious diseases) are now lingering and lurking in hospitals (as one pregnant mother in Orlando, Florida learned when giving birth to her baby; after which she was informed she picked up an infectious virus and must have her arms and legs amputated). So much for the days of happy child birth experiences at hospitals.

Medical interventions that speed up the delivery of babies have been scientifically researched extensively and said to increase the complications of the health of the baby at child birth; among the complications being respiratory problems. Giving mothers pain killers and epidurals can in fact hinder the well-being and health of the baby, by thwarting the natural delivery process, imparting toxic drugs into the mother (and thereby the baby connected at the umbilical cord) and hindering the baby's lung capacity and oxygen intake thereby.

Therefore it is vitally important to guard yourself from unnecessary medical interventions, which may profit the physician, but not you the patient (nor your beloved children and family).

Removing a woman's uterus and ovaries is a questionable practice, as there are far better ways to deal with the underlying problem than to begin removing vital body parts and disrupting a woman's hormones. The same applies to removing a man's testicles (fearing testicular or prostate cancer) as testosterone in actuality helps heat up the body and kill cancer (and other diseases). Moreover testosterone gives men the ability to fight, the will to live and be a man (without which few men want to remain alive).

Testosterone and HGH Injections

Ironically testosterone injections for men over 40 years of age prevents cancer, as testosterone levels decline in men throughout middle age and onward. Thus these absent minded physicians cutting off men's balls (to prevent prostate cancer) could do them more good by giving them testosterone and HGH injections to restore the body's heat, virility, male aggression, blood circulation and burn away the cancer within (the prostate and any other bodily organs). Of course you will need to get testosterone and human growth hormone (HGH) from a medical doctor and pharmacist in the United States, as I have in the past via anti-aging clinics and physicians. When living overseas many pharmacies sell these over the counter, as other governments do not see these substances as harmful as does the FDA (or possibly it's all about control and managing the substance to ensure the right people profit from its manufacture and sale).

Nevertheless HGH helps me sleep better, unlike the damnable sleeping pills my father's evil doctor in Florida gave him for years that fried his brain and gave him Alzheimer's and dementia (all for profit as physicians prey on patients like drug dealers seeking ongoing faithful clients for life). Of course my father refused to listen to me and instead was another one of the millions of prescription drug addicts in the United States of addiction that became ensnared in the pill pushing paradigm of American medicine (sadly), though I earnestly and repeatedly warned him (but he opted to listen to the know it all medical doctors and my stepmother was no use, nor any good at persuading him otherwise either). Thus when my father got on more drugs from the doctors to deal with his Alzheimer's and dementia (so many profitable drugs, well beyond the dosage and various meds he actually needed) he began rapidly losing weight (more than 60 pounds), began falling down, and sitting in the living room chair staring at the walls all day wondering which way was up and whether he was coming or going.

Listen carefully, lest you follow into the same snare of your doctor and become another casualty of American medicine, live weak, die prematurely, and never fulfill your total lifelong purpose and destiny.

Vitamin C and B12 Injections

A former Pastor of mine in southern California always got a B12 injection before traveling internationally to strengthen his immune system. He swore by it and said he had good results. I tried it once and found it made my face a bit puffy and never did it again, choosing instead to occasionally take chewable B12 vitamins.

I have taken vitamin C intravenous injections, administered by a physician, of glutathione (from Italy) and placenta (from Japan) before in Asia with good results. In fact the results were so remarkable not only did I feel energized within, some small skin spots on my arms temporarily disappeared for a few weeks. Thus if I had continued taking the injections regularly on a monthly basis I could greatly improve my skin and remedy some of my blemishes. Placenta when injected in the body, according to the medical doctor from USC and the author of "The End of Illness" (as I heard him speak live on a TV program) alerts the body to produce new cells, as the body doesn't know any difference from a newborn baby and immediately goes to work. HgH has a similar result for me and greatly improves my skin, energy levels and enables me to sleep more deeply and restfully.

All of these collectively play a role in combating and killing cancer. Most importantly, listen to your body, consult a medical doctor (as we are talking about controlled substances not easily obtained without a medical doctor's prescription in most countries), and figure out what works best for you. Yet one thing is for sure, these natural substances (though controlled by physicians) are far more useful than unnatural chemicals used in chemo-"therapy" to supposedly "treat" cancer which tend to kill patients and hasten their funerals.

A fellow teacher who worked with me who was 67 years old (and actually looked like he was in his early 50s) told me he has been taking vitamin C and B injections for 15 years. He actually smokes and drinks alcohol, but still looks amazing. He swears by vitamin C and say he learned it from Linus Pauling (a deceased world renown medical physician). Dr. Mercola, an excellent physician advocating that patients become students of health and take back control of their health, says: "Vitamin C is one of the most well-established traditional antioxidants we know of, and its potent health benefits have been clearly demonstrated over time, especially for the prevention and treatment of infectious diseases."

Mercola wrote an interesting article about Linus Pauling summarizing the following:

Was Linus Pauling Right About Vitamin C's Curative Powers After All?

- One of the most famous forerunners of high dose vitamin C treatment for disease prevention was Dr. Linus Pauling, a biochemist and peace activist, and a two-time Nobel Laureate

- A large, decade-long study found that men who took 800 mg of vitamin C per day had less heart disease and lived up to six years longer than those following the conventional guideline of 60 mg/day

- Vitamin C, when administered intravenously at high doses, has been shown to be selectively cytotoxic against cancer cells

Read it in full here below:

https://articles.mercola.com/sites/articles/archive/2015/11/23/vitamin-c-curative-power.aspx

Oregon State University has a Linus Pauling Institute and Micronutrient Information Center that provides more information about vitamin C and other important vitamins and minerals.

https://lpi.oregonstate.edu/mic/vitamins/vitamin-C

I was utterly shocked every time I saw the 67 year old teacher, because he always looks great and told me he never gets sick (and has good muscle on him too). He told me in confidence he has taken vitamin C and B injections regularly for 15 years with great success.

Increase Oxygen

Here are some powerful supplements to increase your oxygen levels:

1. Lily of the Desert Preservative Free Organic Inner Fillet Aloe Vera Juice, 128 Ounce - Supports Health Digestion

https://amzn.to/2J28ypM

Lily Of The Desert Juice Aloe Vera Pf Whl Lea (32 ounces) - Glass Jar

https://amzn.to/2EOJUDK

2. L-Arginine

/&tag=motispeaforco-20

Respiratory Obstructions

Having lived as a missionary and teacher in China, India, and Thailand (among other countries); I witnessed students habitually coughing (perhaps due to air pollution and also environmental pollution depending on where their parents live). The air we breathe, the water we drink and the food we eat greatly impacts our well being.

Chemical trails were continually being sprayed in the skies of Orlando, Florida (the last 10 years or more I lived there) directly over my home and neighborhood. Yet although my home was in the direct path of commercial airlines flying to and from MCO (airport); the chemical trails I am referring to (crisscrossing the sky overhead and destroying perfectly blue skies in the sunshine state of Florida) were in fact being sprayed by military and military contractor planes conducting environmental experimentation and geo-engineering across America (and many other NATO countries such as France - as I saw the same occur in Paris on a perfectly blue day overhead until a chem trail was sprayed in the sky).

Some allege these chem trails are intended to reduce the temperature in the sky and earth below to prevent global warming or climate change, others speculate they are for the intention of military practices to prepare our nation in the event of a war (so we have an additional advantage with such "technology" to be able to artificially manufacture weather patterns in our nation and others in the event of combat). Universities such as Carnegie Mellon and Harvard have commented on these practices online, the former even hosted an entire conference on the matter of geo-engineering.

Certainly ecocide occurred in Vietnam during the Vietnam War, when American planes sprayed "agent orange" overhead polluting the environment and soil below; resulting in four generations of Vietnamese babies being born with deformities (as I witnessed with my own eyes when traveling throughout Vietnam in 2011 and completing global intensive coursework there with New York University).

Here below are some videos I produced over the years on chemical trails polluting our skies overhead (without giving the citizens below a say or vote in the matter before our governments agreed to and permitted such experimentation to occur in the skies above us, which directly affect the health of us living below them).

Env Health Speaker, Respiratory Problems, Chemtrails Hybrid Parasite

https://www.youtube.com/watch?v=2svcAcCYhaM

Chemtrails Attorney - Chemtrails Lawyer - Chemtrail Health Violations

https://www.youtube.com/watch?v=Tq9N9rOb1IU

Chemtrail Parasites - Air Pollution - Trouble Breathing - Morgellons

https://www.youtube.com/watch?v=pacjai4A5XE

Env Experiments - Vietnam Ecocide - Birth Defects - Chemtrails

https://www.youtube.com/watch?v=8RmDj4mHde

M

Breathing Problems - Trouble Breathing - Chemtrails and Morgellons

https://www.youtube.com/watch?v=8NYX-

kYToXw

Ecocide - Vietnam War - Chemtrails - Public Health Speaker

https://www.youtube.com/watch?v=hYL767p1JfI

Chemtrails, NATO climate engineering, Morgellons parasite

https://www.youtube.com/watch?v=Pcj3nslbOmQ

Public Health Warning - Stop Chemtrails and Geo Engineering

https://www.youtube.com/watch?v=EX-Ih3MRsUA

Chemtrail Parasites - Air Pollution - Trouble Breathing - Morgellons

https://www.youtube.com/watch?v=pacjai4A5XE

Nerve Damage - Paralysis - Chemtrail Morgellon Parasite

https://www.youtube.com/watch?v=y5WrQIaDqQw

Medical doctor Hiromi Shinya, professor at Einstein Medical College in Manhattan, New York was embarrassed and humiliated when his beloved daughter had dermatitis and stomach problems, which he as a physician could not heal, correct, or resolve (as he states in his book "The Enzyme Factor" - http://amzn.to/192i6bM).

It was when this brilliant, resilient and persistent doctor created the colonoscopy to go inside and evaluate the stomachs of patients (he having been inside over 300,000 stomachs including those of celebrities and presidents) that he realized meat and dairy are most harmful to the gut, intestinal lining, cause inflammation and thus can at times hinder breathing and other bodily functions.

One of the best things to drink to remove parasites and rid the gut of Candida and cancerous growths, I have personally found, is drinking aloe (which is more rich in oxygen than anything else you can eat or drink). My favorite aloe juice provider is Lily of the Dessert (from Arizona), which I typically would either buy online or at Whole Foods. I found online was cheaper here (and came in glass jars, which Whole Foods often did not have preferring plastic containers which I'm not a fan of as the plastics can leach into liquid substances).

Cloves, which my grandmother used to put in ham for flavor (possibly cloves were used decades ago to kill parasites when cooking also), when she cooked one for a Sunday dinner; is another useful way to rid the body of parasites. Chew up some cloves and swallow them. It is said they kill parasites (as do grapefruit and pumpkin seeds - being anti-parasitic).

Supplements to Increase Oxygen

- Lily of the Desert Preservative Free Organic Inner Fillet Aloe Vera Juice, 128 Ounce - Supports Health Digestion

https://amzn.to/2J28ypM

Lily Of The Desert Juice Aloe Vera Pf Whl Lea (32 ounces) - Glass Jar

https://amzn.to/2EOJUDK

Remember human beings can only live 2 minutes without oxygen. We can go 2 days without water and 40 days without food. Yet oxygen is so often neglected as the corporations of the world involved in heavy industry and manufacturing continue to use the skies above us as an open sewer (and thereby contaminate the air we all breathe and our water supply due to rainfall containing such hazardous and toxic chemicals from the skies).

My students habitually coughing would disrupt classes and themselves when trying to focus academically. It was then that I began making suggestions to them for helpful dietary supplements and natural remedies I myself take as a teacher living abroad in developing countries to strengthen my human immunity and prevent illness (as schools are common breeding grounds for viruses, bacteria and illnesses), much like prisons (where large groups of people congregate and interact closely).

Liver Cleanse to Detox

If you are overweight, have pain in your internal organs (like within your liver and gallbladder) being junked up and in need of a serious ongoing detox (both to lose weight and to improve your internal organs function and thereby your breathing); I recommend a liver cleanse (via coffee enemas) also called colonics by some nurses and health clinics who administer this to help people repair, decontaminate and break free blockages within their digestive tract (wherein 60% or more of your immune system is found).

I will say this as a note of caution however, the first (and last - as I never did it again with the assistance of someone) colonics I did; afterward I think I slept for 12 hours (quite possibly because it drained my electrolytes and may have been excessive as colonics is done with a machine as opposed to a liver cleanse via a coffee enema or the olive oil and lemon juice combination (which I now do and prefer), the latter options both allow your body to determine naturally how much to remove via the anus - versus a machine with colonics just pulling stuff out of you at its own pace, and quite possibly as I experienced far too much).

I realize not everyone is keen to do such a thing, but if you understood how effective a properly performed liver cleanse is (as I felt 10 years younger and renewed within afterward); you would be less inclined to resist and more focused on the final outcome and improved results and health benefits.

In fact when I did coffee enemas, the first thing I would feel was my ears would open up (as when riding on a plane and ascending to higher altitudes). Although I do not fully understand it, I experientially know it to be true (every time I did a coffee enema - which I did for 2 years or more).

I experienced great results, an increase in energy and reduced internal burden on my body (which consistently comes through a polluted food and water supply, toxic environment in which we live, medicines, stress and so much more than we realize).

Cars get serviced and have oil and fluid changes. Yet human beings going through life never have any of these, which results in an automobile breaking down and ceasing to operate properly after about 10 years in service.

Hereafter I have created some videos to help you capture the essence of the liver, its vital functions, burdensome challenges, and ways to help detoxify your liver and body. These videos were made several years ago. I therefore apologize in advance for them, but not for the profound, enlightening and life-saving information therein. Should you want personalized attention, health coaching and wellness training; please contact me directly to schedule a paid consultation (RevivingNations@yahoo.com).

Detoxification - Liver Cleanse (1 of 2)

https://www.youtube.com/watch?v=hqMlZ0jPt1k

Detoxification - Liver Cleanse (2 of 2)

https://www.youtube.com/watch?v=34u_nBtgU74

Detox FDA Acetaminophen

Meds Drugs Liver Damage

https://www.youtube.com/watch?v=9hQq_L9FX0U

Coffee Cleanse - Coffee Enema (1 of 2)

https://www.youtube.com/watch?v=CdyrjGASHDM

Coffee Cleanse - Coffee Enema (2 of 2)

https://www.youtube.com/watch?v=XLcjw8NHopc

Liver Cleanse - Fatty Liver (1 of 3)

https://www.youtube.com/watch?v=a4LqDQMNKvk

Liver Cleanse - Improve Breathing (2 of 3)

https://www.youtube.com/watch?v=tzKfUVGZ0hE

Health Speaker - Liver Cleanse (3 of 3)

https://www.youtube.com/watch?v=kkNF57HLWAw

Deadly Parasites - Parasite Cleanse

https://www.youtube.com/watch?v=untcwTVG_lo

Health Coach, Wellness Speaker - Liver Cleanse Steps (1of5)

https://www.youtube.com/watch?v=9Vo1s2ZMGaQ

Health Coach, Wellness Speaker - Liver Cleanse Steps (2of5)

https://www.youtube.com/watch?v=sAQiNJCS1Rw&t=1s

Health Coach, Wellness Speaker - Liver Cleanse Steps (3of5)

https://www.youtube.com/watch?v=WsY83FkG_9U

Health Coach, Wellness Speaker - Liver Cleanse Steps (4of5)

https://www.youtube.com/watch?v=PBPyC7t4x-0

Health Coach, Wellness Speaker - Liver Cleanse Steps (5of5)

https://www.youtube.com/watch?v=YTacUg-5G2U

Nutritional Suggestions

Upon talking to an American nurse in China (at the school where I formerly taught) and a chemistry teacher, I discovered during a lunch conversation that raw honey is a natural antibiotic. It was that night when I went to the grocery store next door to my apartment to find the three darkest most pure appearing brands of raw honey I could locate (from China, Europe and Australia) and began taking a teaspoon or a bit more daily; to strengthen my immunity. It truly worked because whenever I felt the slightest scratch in my throat or pain, after taking honey the mucus immediately came out of my throat and I began feeling better.

Dr. Hiromin Shinya is his book "The Enzyme Factor" (http://amzn.to/192i6bM) talks about papaya and pineapple having waste removing enzymes, which I highly recommend you eat regularly to help your body detox and heal itself.

Increase Oxygen

Also I recommend eating and drinking aloe juice (Lily of the Dessert is an excellent brand in the

USA - https://amzn.to/2J28ypM) as aloe is rich in oxygen, which certainly helps increase your oxygen levels and remove cancer in the intestinal tract (where up to 60% of your immune system is found).

L-Arginine is an amino acid that increases nitric oxygen in the blood stream and energizes the body and male libido (https://amzn.to/2tZxe82). I highly recommend it and foods rich in L-Arginine.

Daily exercise (even walking) will improve your circulation, oxygen intake, and respiratory function. Whether you walk to work, outdoors for recreation, with your spouse after work, or to help the old lady across the street; all are good and beneficial (as is going to the local health club and burning fat via sweating on a stair master or treadmill).

Environmental Health

As the cancer villages of China have taught us, where soil is toxic from industrial dumping and disregard of heavy metals and toxic chemicals leaching into the soil and aquifer, consequently to pollute the rice grown therein; consumers of food need to be alert and aware as to WHERE their food comes from, HOW it is grown, WHO is growing it (and their values and motives - profit, sustainable profit, or a quality product to sustain generations with environmental ethics for the ecosystem and all complementary parts).

When Chinese in rural villages began getting sick, eventually they traced their illness to the poor environment in which the rice they were eating was grown. As a result, they stopped eating rice grown in a toxic and polluted environment, but continued to sell the same rice to unsuspecting consumers within the cities of their nation (and likely elsewhere in Asia and beyond to the detriment of the health of unsuspecting consumers, being easy to bypass lazy and uneducated governments' customs officials).

When we continually drink bad water, eat contaminated food, and breathe polluted air; these toxic inputs weaken our immunity and overall health. Medicine will not necessarily remove the toxic environmental inputs into our daily lives, but in fact will increase human toxicity and the burden to our liver, gallbladder and kidneys (vital waste removing organs).

Humans therefore must be alert and aware as to their environment and the impact of negative and toxic influences interfering with our well-being and disrupting the ecosystem in which we as humans live, lest we be unable to continue to survive and thrive.

Ironically, many "air fresheners" and household "cleaning supplies" have toxic petro-chemicals within them that cause leukemia, cancer and many other illnesses in humans. The book "Solvent Neurotoxicity" - http://amzn.to/1hrlGNz (written by a PhD from Denmark) reveals how solvents used to mix various chemicals and concoctions are quite toxic - specifically methyl, ethyl and benz named solvents and substances.

Ten harmful solvents to take note of are: (Chloromethane; Dichloromethane; N-Hexane; Methyl Ethyl Ketone; Methyln N-Butyl Ketone; Styrene; Toluene; 1,1,1-Trichloroethane, Trichloroethylene, and Xylene) and two mixtures of solvents (White Spirit, Mixed solvent exposure) have been selected based on their widespread use, as well as the mounting evidence from research concerning the neurotoxicity of these particular solvents. Evidence from animal and human experiments, clinical observations, and epidemiological studies reveal their toxicity and how harmful they can be to human health.

Health conscious consumers, researchers, occupational hygiene specialists, epidemiologists, trade unions, construction and manufacturing department heads and foremen, along with industry leaders and employees working with organic solvents will find this book to be essential in determining methods for preventing chronic toxic neuropathy, encephalopathy, and other solvent-related disorders.

Just remember the only Benz you want in your life is a Mercedes (car). Otherwise get rid of the rest as benzene, removed from gasoline in the 1970s and reduced to a few parts per billion, causes leukemia and cancer. The U.S. Marine training base in Camp Lejeune found toxic benzene in their water supply, which caused families living on the military base to become very ill (some getting leukemia and cancer before dying and leaving us). The name of the documentary film exposing the incident is named "Semper Fi" (meaning always faithful) and can be seen at the web link hereafter: http://amzn.to/1Bvl2es

Solvent neurotoxicity causes acute and chronic neurotoxicity within humans via a number of harmful solvents commonly used in household cleaning supplies, cosmetics, air fresheners, and volatile chemicals even in car seats (to name just a few). These toxic chemicals can not only disrupt human hormones, but even make a car malfunction (as recently evidenced in the case of Sabaru when toxic perfumes and cleaning agents used therein made brake lights inoperable and defective).

The following articles below document in detail how toxic chemicals, particularly solvents, can impair automobiles and make manufacturing workers ill also.

https://www.caranddriver.com/news/a26595369/sub
aru-recall-impreza-forester-brake-lights/

https://www.ncbi.nlm.nih.gov/pubmed/27737812

https://www.tandfonline.com/doi/abs/10.1080/0963
8280110102126

https://www.ascentforums.com/forum/16-off-topic-
discussion/6597-largest-subaru-recall-ever-brake-
lights.html

The dirty dozen chemicals to watch out for
are indeed ubiquitous and hard to avoid. These
articles will serve as a further resource to perhaps
guide you:

The Ugly Side of the Beauty Industry
https://amzn.to/2tWoz6p

Toxic Relief - Restore Health and Energy

https://amzn.to/2VPnwkF

Dirty Dozen 12 Ingredients to Avoid

http://ecodiscoveries.com/eco-friendly-green-cleaning-products-blog/dirty-dozen-12-ingredients-to-avoid-in-cosmetics-and-5-clean-beauty-brands-to-try/

Dirty Dozen Cosmetic Chemicals to Avoid

https://davidsuzuki.org/queen-of-green/dirty-dozen-cosmetic-chemicals-avoid/

Dirty Dozen 12 Toxic Chemicals in Makeup and Cosmetics You Must Avoid

http://www.alyaka.com/magazine/dirty-dozen-12-toxic-chemicals-makeup-cosmetics-must-avoid/

Vitamins and Mineral Supplements

Zinc is a powerful antioxidant and essential mineral vitally important for prenatal and postnatal development. Zinc deficiency negatively impacts up to two billion people around the world and is attributed to many diseases. Children with an insufficient supply of zinc in their bodies experience growth retardation, delayed sexual maturation, susceptibility to infection, and diarrhea.

I have experienced all of these in that I am not as tall as my father, did not reach puberty until I was 15 years of age, had allergies throughout my teenage years, often got sick when traveling overseas in developing countries, and had nonstop diarrhea in India for two months straight (and several other countries around the world when traveling as a missionary).

Zinc plating is used to reduce corrosion in iron and electrical batteries. Dietary supplements with zinc include zinc carbonate and zinc gluconate. Deodorants use zinc chloride. Anti-dandruff shampoos use zinc pyrithione to prevent dandruff. Excess zinc some believe causes copper deficiency, ataxia, and lethargy.

The world's zinc supply is largely deposited in Australia, Canada and the United States. The largest zinc reserves in the world however are in Iran. Zinc mines are mainly in China, Australia, and Peru.

Next to iron, aluminum, and copper; zinc is the fourth most commonly used metal in the world.

Within dietary supplements, zinc comes in the following forms: zinc oxide, zinc acetate, zinc gluconate, and zinc picolinate.

Zinc deficiency has been associated with major depression. Zinc has been used extensively to treat children with diarrhea in the developing world (as the essential mineral is further depleted during diarrhea). Replenishing the body's zinc for two weeks and supplementing your daily allowance will lessen the likelihood of getting diarrhea or it reoccurring after already having it.

The good news is zinc picolinate (the form I use which is less hard on the stomach and more easily absorbed) is also excellent for improving the respiration of the lungs and thereby our ability to breathe without obstructions.

One study showed taking zinc supplementation reduces the progression of age related macular degeneration, which is to say zinc sustains and strengthens the eyes in humans.

Zinc also improves skin conditions such as dandruff and acrodermatitis enteropathica (a genetic disorder affecting zinc absorption that was fatal to infants). Intranasal sprays use zinc, but when used in excess can reduce a human's sense of smell.

The antimicrobial action of the ions in zinc improve the gastrointestinal tract and function, while also strengthening human immunity. Moreover large amounts of zinc when added to a urine sample, have the ability to mask the detection of drugs.

The inflammation within the nasal passage way during the flu, common cold, and allergy season can be helped and mitigated by zinc. Thus many cold and flu remedies have zinc within them, especially throat lozenges.

My favorite form of zinc is NowFoods zinc picolinate in capsules for easy absorption accessible here: http://amzn.to/1WbrG3M

Taking beyond 75 milligrams a day within a 24 hour timeframe has been found to reduce cold and flu symptoms. By suppressing nasal inflammation, zinc has the ability to inhibit the human rhinovirus from replicating and spreading in the nasal mucosa within the nasal passageway.

Other forms of zinc that typically are less expensive (unlike the zinc picolinate, which I use from NowFoods) can result in nausea and a bad taste in one's mouth.

Topically, zinc oxide protects against sunburns in the summer and windburns in the winter. Likewise zinc oxide can prevent a baby from getting a diaper rash.

https://en.wikipedia.org/wiki/Zinc

More insightful articles with a wealth of information to help you on your journey to improve your breathing (and likely any skin ailments) are here after below.

Zinc and Respiratory Infections

https://www.who.int/elena/titles/zinc_pneumonia_children/en/

The Importance of Zinc in Respiratory Diseases

- https://www.asianscientist.com/2018/01/in-the-lab/lung-disease-zinc-cigarette-smoke/

New insights into the role of zinc in the respiratory epithelium.

https://www.ncbi.nlm.nih.gov/pubmed/11264713

Over the past 30 years, many researchers have demonstrated the critical role of zinc (Zn), in diverse physiological processes, such as growth and development, maintenance and priming of the immune system, and tissue repair. The physiology of zinc and its vital beneficial role in the respiratory epithelium is irrefutable. Zinc diversely acts as: (i) an anti-oxidant; (ii) an organelle stabilizer; (iii) an anti-apopototic agent; (iv) an important cofactor for

DNA synthesis; (v) a vital component for wound healing; and (vi) an anti-inflammatory agent.

Thus zinc is a major dietary anti-oxidant, which has a protective role for the airway epithelium against oxy-radicals and other noxious agents. Zinc therefore has important implications for asthma and other inflammatory diseases where the physical barrier is vulnerable and compromised.

Once again here is the exact link to zinc picolinate to help improve your breathing and the health of your lungs:

http://amzn.to/1WbrG3M

The Great Windkeeper (direct link to buy online below) is another excellent and wonderful natural herbal supplement I learned about from

Chinese acupuncture, which I have used with great results.

https://amzn.to/2IB5wZo

The "Great Windkeeper" seems to be some sort of herbal remedy with plum tea. My experience is it dries up the mucus and cause of inflammation within your gut and lungs. A couple days after I began to use "The Great Windkeeper" my bowel movement was a bit harder and compacted, as whatever was blocking my breathing from within my lungs and nose seemed to have dried up and came out the back end in the toilet like a brick.

Breathing better is truly worth it, as oxygen intake is vitally important for optimal and good health. Remember without oxygen, the human body cannot function and all energy and life within ceases to exist. Cardiopulmonary resuscitation requires ongoing oxygen flow to and through the lungs to strengthen and sustain the body.

Vitamins and Mineral Supplements

One of my favorites and a new discovery is Alpha Lipoic Acid (ALA), which is a naturally occurring antioxidant, quite essential for the functioning of critical enzymes involved in glucose and amino acid metabolism. ALA is a coenzyme and a potent antioxidant. Mitochondria, the energy generators of our cells, use ALA for both protection and to generate vitally important cellular energy. Actively involved in both the water and fatty compartments of cells, ALA fights free radicals throughout the body.

Furthermore ALA promotes healthy blood sugar metabolism alongside a healthy balanced diet, supports mitochondrial energy production, and energizes the body's defense mechanism against free radicals.

Moreover ALA helps recycle antioxidant nutrients such as vitamin C and E vitally important for cancer prevention and healing the skin. As a former lifeguard from Florida, I know the importance of vitamins C and E.

I recommend drinking a lot of water whenever taking supplements as too much of anything can be toxic to your kidneys and/or liver. Like a toilet, your body needs water to flush and remove waste and rid the body of impurities; lest they linger and cause havoc in the body. If you feel like you a pooping bricks; you likely are dehydrated and not drinking enough water and/or lack fiber in your diet (which can easily be obtained by eating more raw fruit and vegetables).

Vitamin C, Glutathione & Placenta

In fact one of the cancer cures that can be pursued naturally is vitamin C injections, along with glutathione and placenta (which I have done with great success several times, witnessing immediate improvements on my skin as pre-cancerous growths temporarily disappeared). Had I remained in the country where I get these injections, I could have done them regularly with prolonged success.

Glutathione is naturally occurring within the liver and the precursor to all energy within the body, being vital for internal detoxification. It is found in many of our tropical fruits, which I highly recommend eating to energize the body and detox your intestinal tract. I've taken intravenous injections of glutathione administered by a physician (which I do NOT recommend any other way, but thru a licensed medical doctor).

Glutathione Supplements (Oral)

Bulletproof Glutathione Force, Master Antioxidant for Detox and Immune Support (90 Capsules)

https://amzn.to/2uCvBh9

As the body's master antioxidant, glutathione is a powerful supplement useful to detoxify the body and support human immunity. Among the many things which deplete glutathione in the body are stress, poor diet, and environmental toxins. Glutathione can lessen, mitigate and help stop the free radical chain reactions occurring in the body (and that result in undigested renegade proteins causing cancer).

Natural Vore Glutathione Supplement - Skin Whitening Anti-Aging Benefits - Pure Antioxidant Milk Thistle Extract Liver Detox

https://amzn.to/2HZ1Tum

Optimized Liposomal Glutathione Softgels NO-Taste | Pure Reduced Glutathione 500mg | Liver Detox, Brain Function | China-Free Setria® Glutathione, Soy-Free Gluten-Free, Dairy Free, Non-GMO

https://amzn.to/2V801mX

Jarrow Formulas Reduced Glutathione, Supports

Liver Health, 500 mg, 120 Veggie caps

https://amzn.to/2UiZvp8

I know I talk tough about doctors and can be
hard on them, but I do respect medical doctors with
pure motives who legitimately do their job and seek
the well-being of their patients (which hopefully
most do, but that is not to say there is not some
wiggle room within which physicians up sell
patients and maneuver subtly to enlarge their profit
margins in a questionable manner). For example
when paying out of pocket, physicians often charge
patients less than when they bill insurance
companies (and often excessively bill insurers).

Dr. Michael Rosin, a Sarasota, Florida licensed dermatologist cut elderly patients countless times, taking biopsies and removing skin lesions he lied and told patients were cancerous; in order to rake in $2,500 a cut via insurance billings by which he financially enriched himself (and made patients suffer physically with lacerations, cuts and scars on various parts of their bodies). Here below CNBC covered the story on their epic show "American Greed":   https://www.cnbc.com/id/100000079

Of course the brilliant and presumptuously almighty United States Food and Drug Administration, which profits handsomely off the drug licenses and permits it issues to drug companies, has not evaluated these statements and will say ALA (and my other recommendations within this book) are not intended to diagnose, treat, cure or prevent any disease. I respect the FDA (and agree to comply with the law) as a legal regulatory agency, despite its ongoing history of corruption and being in bed with the very industries it claims to regulate (as the executives from the very industries in agriculture, food and drugs find their way on to regulatory boards, committees and seats of power to make critical decisions impacting national and global public health).

Milk Thistle

Milk thistle is another great natural liver detox supplement to take. Beware it will make you go to the bathroom a lot, but greatly reduce your body's toxic burden within and truly energize you making you feel like an elementary school kid all over again. Therefore I recommend taking it when you are home at night or over the weekend (or on your days off work in case you need to run to the bathroom).

Pure Milk Thistle Supplement 1000mg - 200 Capsules, Max Strength 4X Concentrated Extract 4:1 Milk Thistle Seed Powder Herb Pills, 1000 mg Silymarin Extract for Liver Support, Cleanse, Detox & Health

https://amzn.to/2uyS7HF

The liver plays an important role in the body removing harmful waste and toxins, among 1,000 other vital functions all interrelated. Milk Thistle supports liver function and health, being a powerful antioxidant, free radical scavenger and detoxifier advancing the removal of harmful toxins from the body. Milk Thistle thereby promotes heart health, balanced cholesterol levels, and has anti-aging benefits.

Organic Milk Thistle Capsules, 1500mg 4X Concentrated Extract is the Strongest Milk Thistle Supplement Available. Silymarin is Great for Liver Cleanse & Detox! 120 Vegetarian Capsules

https://amzn.to/2HOMcH2

As for me, given that I have had skin issues on my body, some which one dermatologist in New York City (Spring Street Dermatology) wanted to cut for profit (along with some other useless but profitable procedures that were performed on me to correct a skin problem on my face, which since improved without her help when I changed my diet, began taking certain health supplements mentioned in this book, and stopped wearing briefs and switched to boxers so my body is not overheating internally).

After having bought thousands of dollars of books on cancer, microbiology, parasite cleanses, health, wellness and detoxification; I have relentlessly studied this topic for years (while practicing with my own body using a plant based diet, coffee enemas, and certain supplements) and learned some important things about cancer.

Putrefaction pathways of undigested proteins results in harmful bacteria populating the gut within the intestines, polluting the colon, and can eventually lead to colorectal and other cancers. As we age into adulthood, the body produces fewer vitally important enzymes to aid food digestion and absorption; resulting in runaway undigested proteins causing havoc within the body (particularly those coming from meat and dairy products).

I want you to know I eat meat and dairy (most only yogurt as for dairy, perhaps occasionally cheese a few times a year when eating pizza or baked goods). I prefer goat cheese when possible, but cannot lie I also enjoy swizz and mozzarella cheese (occasionally on my eggs). When at the Eiffel Tower, I will probably enjoy a ham and cheese crepe. Yet not everything that tastes good going down is easily digested in your stomach.

To help with this process I recommend digestive enzymes and Alpha Lipoic Acid (ALA).

Digestive Enzymes

Source Naturals Essential Enzymes

500mg Bio-Aligned Multiple Enzyme Supplement

Herbal Defense For Digestion, Gas, Constipation &

Bloating Relief - Supports A Strong Immune

System - 240 Capsules

https://amzn.to/2FKCN15

Pure Encapsulations - Digestive Enzymes

Ultra - Comprehensive Blend of Vegetarian

Digestive Enzymes - 90 Capsules

https://amzn.to/2I1BuMy

Alpha-Lipoic Acid

Doctor's Best Alpha-Lipoic Acid, Non-GMO,

Gluten Free, Vegan, Soy Free, Promotes Healthy

Blood Sugar, 600 mg

https://amzn.to/2FQeX2P

Pure Encapsulations - Alpha Lipoic Acid 200 mg -

Hypoallergenic Water- and Lipid-Soluble

Antioxidant Supplement - 60 Capsules

https://amzn.to/2HNZHa2

Renegade Proteins Causing Cancer

The importance of Alpha-Lipoic Acid to metabolize protein (and undigested renegade proteins in the body causing cancer) should not be underestimated.

Here below are some articles on the topic of undigested renegade proteins causing havoc in the body and researchers' latest discoveries, further inquiries, pursuit of knowledge on this important topic, and quest for more information to discover how to combat these proteins gone rogue.

In Silico Analysis of Putrefaction Pathways in Bacteria and Its Implication in Colorectal Cancer.

U.S. National Library of Medicine and National Institutes of Health

https://www.ncbi.nlm.nih.gov/pubmed/29163445

"Fermentation of undigested proteins in human gastrointestinal tract (gut) by the resident microbiota, a process called bacterial putrefaction, can sometimes disrupt the gut homeostasis. In this process, essential amino acids (histidine, tryptophan) that are required by the host may be utilized by the gut microbes. In addition, some of the products of putrefaction, like ammonia, putrescine, cresol, indole, phenol, etc., have been implicated in the disease pathogenesis of colorectal cancer (CRC)" [Putrefaction Pathways, article and web link above].

Maybe my body needs more tryptophan? Interestingly tryptophan is said to be found in turkey, which after eating some claim makes us more sleepy. Of course it is easier to pull away to the bedroom and sleep on Thanksgiving after eating turkey if your distant relatives who suddenly show up at your home are annoying and not interesting to be around (something my paternal grandfather was known to do after a holiday meal). Nevertheless being born the Friday morning after Thanksgiving, turkey and cranberry sauce are among my favorites. I could probably eat a turkey dinner two or three times a week quite happily.

Perhaps this is because my body needs tryptophan for some reason. This is a topic I should further research and investigate when I have time (based on the preceding paragraph that mentioned and brought tryptophan up calling it an essential amino acid. The importance of amino acids to hair, muscular growth and cellular reproduction should not be discounted. I therefore do not advocate (nor belittle) vegetarianism, as I realize the struggle and great difficulty involved (as a former vegetarian for about 2 years and vegan for maybe 1 year) in obtaining and consuming a sufficient amount of protein via a plant based diet (though some like Dr.

Colin Campbell at Cornell University and others, all whom I greatly respect and value their contributions to health and wellness, say otherwise).

Eating is a personal decision; it being done based on appetite, for personal health, and pleasure. Therefore as a body builder into lifting weights to build muscle, I prefer a well balanced diet that includes lean meat, chicken and some fish. My belief is if consumed in moderation, all things on earth are worthy of being thankful for and eating when desirable (Philippians 4:5; 1Timothy 4:4). After the resurrection of Christ, Jesus asked for meat (Luke 24:41; John 21:5) and God told the apostle Peter in a vision to "kill and eat" (Acts 10:13). Therefore like my late friend, chef and travel writer Anthony Bourdain, I agree there is something special in eating a little (or a lot of) meat.

However if you were a gluttonous carnivore for two or three decades, moderation for you (Biblically advisable - Philippians 4:5) may be to try vegetarianism for a few years to cleanse your liver and internal organs, revitalize your body, give your intestines a break from having to digest, assimilate and eliminate all that meat. I suggest pursuing and receiving wise counsel in all things (this book being one way to do that among others) and in the end listening to your body (as it ultimately knows and will tell and signal to you what is best for you).

Bacterial putrefaction pathways associated with such metabolites are therefore of great importance, because this is where the breakdown of the body begins and the decline in human immunity and health occurs. "The majority of bacteria commonly found in the human gut include *Bacillus, Clostridium, Enterobacter, Escherichia, Fusobacterium, Salmonella*, etc. Interestingly, while pathogens utilize almost all the analyzed pathways, commensals prefer putrescine and H2S production pathways for metabolizing the undigested proteins" [Putrefaction Pathways, article and web link above]. The putrefaction pathways in the gut microbiomes of carcinoma (cancer) patients show a higher abundance of putrefying bacteria.

Scrub, Cleanse and Intestinal Detox

One of my favorite concoctions and simple smoothie recipes to scrub, cleanse and detox my body from top to bottom (specifically my entire intestinal tract) is taking an organic lemon and pure high quality apple juice (without sugar or water) and cutting an organic lemon up (with its peel on it, after having washed it) and blending the apple juice and organic lemon together in a smoothie. Upon drinking this the malic acid within apple juice opens the body's bile ducts to detox and remove liver and gallbladder stones, while the lemon fiber and juice scrub your intestinal lining removing candida and cancerous putrefying undigested protein and substances in the body.

I've visually witnessed and seen in my stool in the toilet white Candida appearing slime and mucus, after it has left my body (both after drinking this smoothie and/or after having done a coffee cleanse via an enema).

Dr. Simoncini in Italy believes cancer is a fungus and is white in color. I agree with Simoncini and liken cancer to Candida. Simoncini's book "Cancer Is A Fungus" can be obtained here:

http://amzn.to/1fRx6sG

Some interesting articles (excerpts) and resources about the interaction between protein and gut microbes relevant to intestinal health are here below to further read and explore.

Contributions of the Interaction Between Dietary Protein and Gut Microbiota to Intestinal Health.
U.S. National Library of Medicine and National Institutes of Health

https://www.ncbi.nlm.nih.gov/pubmed/28215168

"There is growing recognition that composition and metabolic activity of the gut microbiota can be modulated by the dietary proteins which in turn impact health. The amino acid composition and digestibility of proteins, which are influenced by its source and amount of intake, play a pivotal role in determining the microbiota. Reciprocally, it appears that the gut microbiota is also able to affect protein metabolism which gives rise to the view that function between the microbiota and protein can proceed in both directions. In response to the alterations in dietary protein components, there are significant changes in the microbial metabolites including short chain fatty acids (SCFAs), ammonia, amines, gases such as hydrogen, sulfide and methane which are cytotoxins, genotoxins and carcinogens associated with development of colon cancer and inflammatory bowel diseases" (Dietary Protein - Intestinal Health).

Evidence clearly suggests "that excessive protein intake adversely affects health. Supplying high and undigested proteins will encourage pathogens and protein-fermenting bacteria to increase the risk of diseases. These changes of microbiota can affect the gut barrier and the immune system by regulating gene expression in relevant signaling pathways and by regulating the secretion of metabolites. ...Attention should be given to the dietary strategies with judicious selection of source and supplementation of dietary protein to benefit gut health" (Dietary Protein - Intestinal Health).

Interesting Articles To Read

- Genetic Assays -

ww.google.com/patents/CN105555972A?cl=en

"In some cases, the first epitope is present in the hemagglutinin **protein** of the ..... **tumor** herpesvirus, poxvirus), the ssDNA virus (+ strand or "sense"), the DNA (For ...... 18B) a further **number** of **undigested DNA** sample may indicate the wrong and ...... through nucleotide sequencing of the p54, p72, and pB602L (CVR) genes."

After Devastating China, African Swine Fever Threatens to Go Global

☐

Swine fever has spread from pigs in Africa to hogs in China and according to epidemiologists is expected to infect the global food supply soon once it spreads to Europe and the Americas (North and South America), as China is one of the world's largest pork suppliers.

Such foodborne diseases explain why many Jews, Muslims and a few smart Christians avoid eating pigs and follow God's dietary guidelines in the Bible. I myself am less frigid and have eaten pork baby back ribs, bacon, and pulled pork burritos happily (just praying over my food and ensuring the restaurants I eat at are reputable and fully cook the meat). Yet I truly should be more cautious since when I was in Malaysia in the late 1990s the government commissioned the military to shoot and kill millions of pigs infected with Japanese encephalitis.

Books and Articles on Food Safety and Health

THE FUTURE OF FOOD - Global Reform to Improve the Quality of Food & Public Health - http://amzn.to/1kcjnUs

THE FUTURE OF FOOD - GMOs, Bogus Science, Agroterrorism and Regulatory Reform
http://amzn.to/1TtOskf

GEOSTRATEGY to Protect Environmental Health and Food Security
http://amzn.to/1BiABrh

Prescription For Nutritional Healing
https://amzn.to/2PzDZay

.

Dead Doctors Don't Lie
https://amzn.to/2XQrmuG

Toxic Relief
https://amzn.to/2XU8TO5

How Doctors Think
https://amzn.to/2VuFZq2

Email me if you want me to speak for you
on disease prevention in your city, state and nation.
(RevivingNations@yahoo.com)
www.PaulFDavis.com

Dhh1p Crystal Structure and Functional Analysis of DEAD-Box Protein

lsi.zju.edu.cn/_upload/article/files/.../7b6d8c74-07dd-4c71-90a5-6c9575678cf9.pdf

"...mammals (RCK/**p54**) has been implicated in certain **tumor** a29209 ... Despite the large **number** of DEAD-box **proteins** from ...... The position of the **undigested**."

Protein Folding, Protein Homeostasis & Cancer

https://www.ncbi.nlm.nih.gov/pmc/articles/PMC40 13342/

"Proteins fold into their functional 3-dimensional structures from a linear amino acid sequence. *In vitro* this process is spontaneous; while *in vivo* it is orchestrated by a specialized set of proteins, called chaperones. Protein folding is an ongoing cellular process, as cellular proteins constantly undergo synthesis and degradation." Here emerging links between this process and cancer occur.

"Citing statistics from the American Cancer Society, Harold Varmus noted that we have made depressingly little progress in combating cancer. While over the past 50 years dramatic strides have been made against cardiovascular and infectious diseases, age-adjusted mortality in patients with cancer has declined only slightly, with the decrease mostly related to the drop in lung cancer-caused deaths due to aggressive efforts to discourage cigarette smoking" (Protein Folding).

Doctors and oncologists continued reliance on chemotherapy and radiation to combat cancer have been fruitless at strengthening patients' human immunity to fight back and combat the disease themselves internally. Thus little progress is being made in cancer prevention and cancer cures from the perspective of traditional medicine and protocols.

Whitesell and Lindquist assert "cancer cells acquire a hyper-mutating phenotype and further claim that control of cancer will best be achieved by modulating cells' ability to adapt and evolve in response to selection pressures" (Protein Folding).

One thing worth noting and remembering is proteostasis (protein homeostasis) as "proteins within in a cell are constantly undergoing renewal, as proteins are degraded and synthesized anew. As proteins are synthesized, they must fold properly to acquire their native, functional form (pathway 1). When this protein folding process misfunctions, misfolded proteins arise (pathway 2). Misfolded proteins may either eventually be converted into properly folded proteins (pathway 3) or be degraded (pathway 4). Native, functional proteins can either spontaneously misfold or undergo degradation (unlabeled pathways)" (Protein Folding).

It is not sufficient to "focus purely on the genotype—we must also understand the means by which the phenotype results from the genotype, both in the cases where the genotype is normal and in those cases where the genotype has undergone changes that characteristic of cancer. Protein folding and proteostasis are the central mechanisms by which the phenotype emerges from the genotype" (Protein Folding).

Heat, Health and Disease Prevention

Dr. Hiromi Shinya, co-creator of the colonoscopy who has been inside 300,000 stomachs (including the guts belonging to celebrities and presidents) and professor at Einstein Medical College in New York, says in his book "Enzyme Factor" that heat stimulates enzymes within the body. This explains why the elderly do better in Florida and living in other warmer places near the equator as they age.

I myself noticed whenever I got sick, a cold, or feverish; by wrapping myself in blankets or bundling up in warm clothes, I can quickly burn away all unwanted bacteria, diseases and viruses and quickly recover. Heat is a powerful force, which is used in food safety to kill salmonella in meat and E. coli in eggs. Likewise your body and immune system benefit from some heat.

Enzyme Factor

Dr. Hiromi Shinya's outstanding book the "Enzyme Factor" is a must read for health conscious people seeking to detoxify their bodies.

http://amzn.to/1f5f7ym

"Christian Anfinsen shared the 1972 Nobel Prize in Chemistry for his work on protein folding. His Nobel lecture, 'Studies on the principles that govern the folding of protein chains', succinctly describes conclusions that set the paradigm for *in vitro* protein folding to this day. With a modest increase in temperature, a protein will lose its original 3D structure but will recover it when the temperature returns to normal. With modest increases in temperature (1°C–2°C), this mild denaturation is reversible. At extremely high temperatures, however, this conformation will turn into a random set of conformations, and it may not revert to the original 3D structure because of denaturation (as in cooking an egg)." [Protein Folding]

Drinking cold drinks during and after meals is therefore not advisable (as it hinders internal body heat and disrupts the digestion, absorption, assimilation and elimination process within the intestines). The older Chinese (as I know from having lived in Taiwan, Hong Kong and mainland China) typically don't drink cold drinks and preferably drink warm water or tea. As I mentioned earlier heat is helpful to combat viruses and diseases (cancer often being linked to undigested proteins which can be reversed in high temperatures), heat being stimulated and achieved by bundling up (jackets or blankets), saunas, living in warm climates, exercise, and/or eating ginger or garlic to help heat up the body and stimulate circulation.

Also for older women estrogen injections and for older men testosterone injections can help stimulate body heat and libido. Ask an anti-aging doctor or health clinic to help you access these after blood work is done to ensure you are able and ready.

"Protein folding *in vivo* is quite different from that *in vitro*. For medium-to-large-sized proteins it occurs much faster than one might expect, typically in the range of milliseconds to seconds. It takes place in the crowded internal environment of the cell, where many intermolecular interactions could potentially disrupt the normal protein folding pathway. Protein folding *in vivo* is facilitated by chaperones, also known as HSPs or stress proteins" (Protein Folding).

Pelham's model "proposes that during heat shock, proteins become partially denatured, exposing hydrophobic regions which then interact to form insoluble aggregates. By binding tightly to hydrophobic surfaces, HSP70 limits such interactions and promotes disaggregation" (Protein Folding).

Historically cancer was said to arise from changes in the DNA sequence of the genomes of cancer cells. An alternative focuses "on the dynamic cellular processes centered on the proteome, and the process of proteostasis" - as "chaperones and protein homeostasis likely play an important role in cancer formation, and thus, present multiple opportunities for therapeutic intervention" (Protein Folding).

It is wise therefore to "search for other overlaps between the heat shock response and virus-induced neoplastic transformation", a suggestion that was not immediately embraced (Protein Folding).

Gerald Krystal, Phd: The Effects of Protein and Carbohydrates on Cancer

https://www.ncbi.nlm.nih.gov/pmc/articles/PMC45 66461/

Purification of a Tyrosine-specific Protein Kinase from Rous Sarcoma Virus-induced Rat Tumor

The Journal of Biological Chemistry

http://www.jbc.org/content/257/12/7135.full.pdf

Crystal Structure and Functional Analysis of DEAD-Box Protein Dhh1p

http://lsi.zju.edu.cn/_upload/article/files/d5/51/7fa6 d96844ce87f6e644da6f67c2/7b6d8c74-07dd-4c71-90a5-6c9575678cf9.pdf

7 Ways Animal Protein is Damaging Your Health

By Sofia Pineda Ochoa, MD, December 31, 2016

https://www.forksoverknives.com/animalproteindan gers/#gs.3m6aj9

Animal Protein and TMAO

"Consuming animal protein results in us having higher circulating levels of trimethylamine N-oxide (TMAO).TMAO is a substance that injures the lining of our vessels, creates inflammation, and facilitates the formation of cholesterol plaques in our blood vessels. And that, of course, is highly problematic for cardiovascular health."

"TMAO is created by complex interactions involving our gut flora and the nutrients in the food we eat. And when we eat animal foods, it alters our gut flora in such a way that facilitates the creation of TMAO."

"So, consuming animal foods result in higher TMAO levels, which is damaging to our vessels. Even without all of the other problematic aspects of animal foods, this one issue involving TMAO is, according to the recent president of the American College of Cardiology Dr. Kim A. Williams, sufficient by itself for people to vigorously avoid animal foods."

Animal Protein and Phosphorus

"Animal protein contains high levels of phosphorus. And when we consume high amounts of phosphorus, one of the ways our bodies normalize the level of phosphorus is with a hormone called fibroblast growth factor 23 (FGF23)," which "has been found to be harmful to our blood vessels. It can also lead to hypertrophy of the cardiac ventricle (abnormal enlargement of our cardiac muscle) and is associated with heart attacks, sudden death, and heart failure. So eating animal protein with its high concentration of phosphorus can result in increased levels of this hormone in our bodies, which in turn is highly problematic for our health."

Animal Protein, Heme Iron and Free Radicals

"Iron is the most abundant metal in the human body. We can consume it in two forms: (a) heme iron, found widely in animal foods like meat, poultry, and fish; and (b) non-heme iron found widely in plant foods."

"One of the problems with heme iron is that it can convert less reactive oxidants into highly reactive free radicals. And free radicals can damage different cell structures like proteins, membranes, and DNA."

"Heme iron can also catalyze the formation of N-nitroso compounds in our bodies, which are potent carcinogens. So, not surprisingly, high intake of heme iron has been associated with many kinds of gastrointestinal cancers as well as other pathologies."

"It is true that heme iron has higher absorption rates and bioavailability than non-heme iron. However, iron itself can cause oxidative stress and DNA damage, so with iron generally, it's not always a situation where "more is better.""

"While we definitely need iron, the absorption and bioavailability of iron from a well-rounded plant-based diet is generally adequate, and we can avoid the problems associated with heme iron and other negative health attributes of animal foods."

What Causes Undigested Food in Stool

https://www.medicalnewstoday.com/articles/321755.php

Various medical conditions "can result in whole or partially digested food in the stool. In these cases, a person often notices other symptoms, such as diarrhea or stomach pain."

"Medical conditions that can cause undigested food to appear in the stool include:"

- **Crohn's disease** - "a type of inflammatory bowel disease that causes inflammation in the digestive tract that can lead to severe diarrhea, abdominal pain, and malnutrition."

- **Celiac disease** - "an autoimmune disorder where the body cannot digest the protein known as gluten that is found in wheat, barley, and certain other grains."

- **Pancreatic insufficiency.** "If a person has a pancreatic insufficiency, they lack enzymes in the pancreas, which leads to the inability to break food down."

- **Lactose intolerance.** "If a person's digestive system is unable to break down the protein in milk and dairy, it may indicate lactose intolerance."

- **Irritable bowel syndrome (IBS).** "IBS is a common condition that affects the large intestine and causes bloating, pain, diarrhea, or constipation. A stomach bug, or gastrointestinal virus, may also cause undigested food in the stool due to food passing quickly through a person's system. Other symptoms of a stomach bug include:"

- fever

- bloating

- abdominal cramping

- diarrhea

- vomiting

- nausea

- body aches

- malaise, or a general feeling of being unwell

Red Meat and Colon Cancer

https://www.health.harvard.edu/newsletter_article/red-meat-and-colon-cancer

"Diet has a powerful influence on many diseases, including America's number two killer, cancer. But because cancer is so complex, with many genetic and environmental factors affecting risk, the link between your menu and your risk has been hard to decipher. In the case of red meat and colon cancer, however, new research provides a plausible explanation for a long-suspected association."

"...Studies from around the world have suggested that a high consumption of meat is linked to an increased risk of colon cancer. In some studies, fresh meat appears culpable; in others, it's processed, cured, or salted meat — but in all cases the worry is confined to red meat, not chicken."

A "study from England showed that large amounts of red meat can produce genetic damage to colon cells in just a few weeks. It's an important finding, but it does not prove that red meat causes cancer. None of the cells were malignant, and the body has a series of mechanisms to repair damaged DNA. In most cases, the repairs are successful, but when they fail, cells can undergo malignant transformation."

In the case of colon cancer, minimize and eat red meat sparingly (a smaller high quality fillet mignon over larger cuts of meat, choose leaner cuts, trim away excess fat, avoid charring your meat on a grill and say no to processed, cured and highly salted meats), keep your caloric intake reasonable, and exercise regularly. "Substitute fish, chicken or turkey (without the skin) for red meat as your main protein source, and experiment with beans as a source of protein, fiber, and vitamins."

A Low-Carb Diet Kills Tumor Cells with a Mutant p53 Tumor Suppressor Gene

The Atkins diet suppresses tumor growth

https://www.ncbi.nlm.nih.gov/pmc/articles/PMC36 10718/

p53 and Its Downstream Proteins as Molecular Targets of Cancer.

https://www.ncbi.nlm.nih.gov/pubmed/16652354

"The p53 tumor suppressor gene plays a key role in prevention of tumor formation through transcriptional dependent and independent mechanisms. Transcriptional-dependent mechanisms are mainly mediated by p53 regulation of downstream targets, leading to growth arrest and apoptosis. Mutational inactivation of the p53 gene is detected in more than 50% of human cancers. Mutation of p53 renders cancer cells more resistant to current cancer therapies due to lack of p53-mediated apoptosis."

The p53 tumor suppressor protein

https://www.ncbi.nlm.nih.gov/books/NBK22268/

"The p53 gene like the Rb gene, is a tumor suppressor gene, i.e., its activity stops the formation of tumors. If a person inherits only one functional copy of the p53 gene from their parents, they are predisposed to cancer and usually develop several independent tumors in a variety of tissues in early adulthood. This condition is rare, and is known as Li-Fraumeni syndrome. However, mutations in p53 are found in most tumor types, and so contribute to the complex network of molecular events leading to tumor formation."

"The p53 gene has been mapped to chromosome 17. In the cell, p53 protein binds DNA, which in turn stimulates another gene to produce a protein called p21 that interacts with a cell division-stimulating protein (cdk2). When p21 is complexed with cdk2 the cell cannot pass through to the next stage of cell division. Mutant p53 can no longer bind DNA in an effective way, and as a consequence the p21 protein is not made available to act as the 'stop signal' for cell division. Thus cells divide uncontrollably, and form tumors."

"Help with unraveling the molecular mechanisms of cancerous growth has come from the use of mice as models for human cancer, in which powerful 'gene knockout' techniques can be used. The amount of information that exists on all aspects of p53 normal function and mutant expression in human cancers is now vast, reflecting its key role in the pathogenesis of human cancers. It is clear that p53 is just one component of a network of events that culminate in tumor formation."

Spring or Alkaline Water

You cannot flush a toilet without water. Likewise you cannot clean a bathtub or sink without water. Therefore when seeking to cleanse and detoxify your body of a cold, flu and disease such as cancer; it is equally important to drink a lot of quality water to flush, wash and cleanse your body from the inside out.

I do not think mineral water is good for the kidneys and prefer either spring water (from a reputable source and NEVER drink Nestle bottled water or water that tastes heavy with metals) or alkaline water (the latter being high in Ph to combat excessive acidity in the body from the typical high protein acidic diet many burden their bodies with). My favorite alkaline water is here below:

Alkaline 88 Bottled Water

https://amzn.to/2FKqIIX

Green Tea

My former dermatologist in New York City who deals with a lot of cancer patients, herself did some research on the topic and found green tea to have anti-cancer fighting properties that is useful for cancer patients to consume.

Be smart and proactive to exercise discretion with the fork, move your body vigorously and happily regularly (walking, bicycling, swimming, boxing, etc.) to burn calories and eliminate toxins, and wash your body thoroughly from within to win the battle against cancer.

When you are not hungry, do not eat (especially in the evening after 6pm if you can avoid doing so - unless you work during the evenings and have an unusual employment schedule). Dr. Hiromi Shinya says fasting is healthy and good for the body, stimulating enzymes within. Likewise I know fasting starves cancer cells in the body and gives your body's organs and cells time to rest and recover from their endless functions, food digestion and transportation of nutrients and minerals throughout the body just being one of many roles and jobs.

Doctors, I am not against you, but rather I am for health and wellness. If it takes people temporarily firing their physician to enable them to take back their health and be responsible to heal their bodies from the inside out - so be it. It is time patients use doctors and stop letting doctors use patients for profit. Once patients understand the foundations of good health and wellness (body, mind and spirit); they then can be more alert, aware and proactive in cultivating a healthy lifestyle (and if necessary occasionally and intelligently pursue the process of hiring a doctor - for a specific purpose) versus always leaning on a physician to sustain them (the latter type of patients often being fragile mentally and emotionally due to their deep dependence on their doctors).

Prayer for Health, Healing and Wellness

The Word of God is life (John 6:63) and also strengthens and energizes the body, the power of the resurrection in Jesus Christ by the Holy Spirit that raised Him from the dead will also bring life and health to your mortal body (Romans 8:11).

Please pray with me now out loud saying:

"Dear Jesus, thank you for dying for me. Come by the power of the Holy Spirit that rose You from the dead and live big in me. Make my life and health what it ought to be. Restore me physically, mentally, emotionally, and spiritually to make me whole. Heal me wonderful Jesus by your supernatural power this very hour. Come blessed Holy Spirit of the living God to comfort (John 14:26) and heal me in the midst of my bodily ailments and weaknesses (Romans 8:26-27). Remove my pain and suffering, causing me to dwell, abide and live daily in divine health. Heal me now in Jesus Name and impart newness of life to me for which I shall give you all the glory. Thank you dear God. Amen."

Upon praying this prayer if you felt the touch of God, supernatural fire (Luke 3:16), a quickening internally and/or physically; I'd love to hear from you.

Know assuredly God is for you and if He be for you nothing can stand against you (Romans 8). Know for sure, it is God's will in Christ Jesus to heal and deliver you so you can be well and whole (read Isaiah 53). Jesus did not only die for humanity's sins and iniquities on the cross, He also died for us to be healed physically and experience newness of life (Romans 6:4; 2Corinthians 5:17).

Surely God Almighty has new life, a better life, a divine breakthrough, healing, restoration and deliverance to energize and empower you physically to enable you to live strong and purposefully to fulfill your divine destiny to give

Him glory as your present battle and test is miraculously transformed and turned into a testimony to bring God honor and glory.

Paul F. Davis is a Wellness Trainer (a former Lifeguard and Personal Fitness Trainer) who has earned 4 Master degrees with honors from the University of Alabama (Health), Michigan State College of Law (Global Food Law), the University of Texas (Educational Leadership), and New York University (Global Affairs). Paul also completed his training in University and Career Counseling at the University of California Los Angeles.

As a Worldwide Motivational Speaker and Travel Writer, Paul has touched 89 nations speaking for the U.S. Military, Companies, Cruise Lines at Sea, Colleges and Universities throughout the globe. Paul is the Author of more than 70 Books on topics ranging from food, health, dating, relationships, international relations, spirituality, the supernatural, empowerment and wealth creation.

Some of Paul's 70+ books include:

- Breathe Better
- The Future of Food (volumes 1 & 2)
- Geostrategy to Protect Environmental Health &
    Food Security
- Breakthrough For A Broken Heart
- Update Your Identity
- Integrity of Heart
- Educational Leadership and School Instruction
- Charter Schools: Faith and Free Choice
- United States of Arrogance
- Healthy Relationships
- Dating, Relationships, Love and Marriage
- God vs. Religion
- Supernatural Fire
- Waves of God
- Empowering & Liberating Women
- College Admissions
- College Advice
- College Match & Self-Discovery
- College Orientation

Many more books and videos can be seen at Paul's website below. Please also connect with Paul via social media. Email Paul for life and health coaching, or college and career counseling.

www.PaulFDavis.com

www.EducationPro.us

www.Linkedin.com/in/worldproperties

www.Facebook.com/speakers4inspiration

www.Twitter.com/PaulFDavis

RevivingNations@yahoo.com

Printed in Great Britain
by Amazon

80697317R00109